*Let Food be thy Medicine
and let Medicine
be thy Food*

HIPPOCRATES

AVD

the anti-viral diet

LIVING TIME™ Books
livingtimebooks.com

AVD

the anti-viral diet

BASED ON THE RESULTS OF RECENT SCIENTIFIC AND MEDICAL RESEARCH

COVID-19 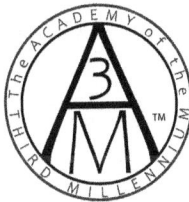 EDITION

Edouard d'Araille

livingtimebooks™

DEDICATED
TO ALL THOSE
WHO ARE READY
FOR CHANGE

the anti-viral diet

AVD is a 'diet book' of a different kind. – Its main aim is not to help you lose weight, counter diabetes, go vegan, clear your mind or eat the best food to support a specific fitness regime. The focus of this new diet is set out in the title alone. Its key purpose is to teach you what food and drink – based on the results of scientific research – are the most likely to protect you from viruses and viral illnesses.

There are, indeed, a number of diets which provide information and advice on what to eat in order to attain *a better state of health*. None of those diets are being dismissed or ignored here. Several of them provide very valuable answers about the effects of diet on your body and a lot of solid practical advice. However, for the purpose of providing clear and unambiguous guidelines on which dietary elements may be most potent as anti-viral agents, this book limits its scope to that topic alone.

AVD is based upon findings from over fifty years of medical research into the effects of various dietary ingredients on viruses and the human immune system. This is not to say that earlier knowledge of diet and medicine – dating back to the Sumerians and the Egyptians – shall be ignored. In fact, a number of dietary elements are included whose benefits were known of a full five thousand years ago. Even in 2nd Millennium BCE Cairo there were at least 850 identified medicines, some still in clinical use.

In this book, 52 biologically active compounds in food and drink – with anti-viral effects – are pinpointed. In some cases, the ingredients may have a direct effect on viruses attacking us – in other cases it is the way in which the ingredients improve responses of our immune system, that may provide us with better protection from viruses.

The book **AVD** presents the results of a review of 50 years of research into the anti-viral effects of dietary ingredients. The work of more than 1000 scientists is represented here. It is stage one of a 3-stage research project initiated by THE ACADEMY OF THE THIRD MILLENNIUM, whose aim is to verify whether an 'anti-viral diet' is a valid, viable hypothesis.

This study is divided into three parts, which progressively present proven data about natural anti-viral agents and how they might serve us in a diet: **Part 1** reflects on our current situation and shares the views of a number of scientists in regard to the usage of natural chemicals in order to defeat viruses. **Part 2** provides core knowledge about the anti-viral and immuno-modulatory properties of fifty-two natural ingredients - all found in food. Substantial research dossiers are provided for each of them, with links to many experiments, studies, reviews, trials and analyses - evidence that supports their inclusion here. Finally, **Part 3** explains in outline a preliminary Anti-Viral Diet with which to incorporate ingredients from Part 2 into one's daily intake. - With this edition, full research dossiers on each ingredient can be accessed by visiting the link at the end of each ingredient section in Part 2. By setting up a free account at https://theantiviraldiet.com you will have life-long access to the ever-increasing database of research which corroborates the validity of an *anti-viral diet*.

We wish to emphasize here that **AVD** is an attempt to arrive at a diet that has broad anti-viral effects and it has not solely been devised with SARS-CoV-2 in mind. The need for us to find effective protection against **all** harmful viruses is a pressing one, as new and dangerous strains - even of known viruses - can wreak such havoc globally. It is hoped that the publication of this study will be of help.

The Academy of the Third Millennium

PAGEFINDER

AVD
the anti-viral diet

PART 1

A NEW DIET

PART 2

the anti-viral diet

52 <u>AVD</u> Ingredients

VITAMINS

MINERALS

NUTRIENTS

FLAVONOIDS

HERBS & SPICES

PLANTS & FLOWERS

GASTRO-MODULATORS

OTHER PHYTOCHEMICALS

PART 3

CREATING YOUR DIET

ACKNOWLEDGEMENTS

__AVD__ is based upon scientific research into natural anti-viral agents and immunomodulatory substances spanning from the 1960s to 2020. It is impossible to pay tribute to all of the researchers and authors who have contributed to advance in the understanding of viruses, anti-viral substances, the human immune system and all of the biochemistry and biogenetics involved in this. The groundbase of research that has been conducted in fields of Immunology, Virology, Infectious Diseases, Pharmaceuticals, Phytochemistry and Human Nutrition over the past half-century - naming only half a dozen areas of relevance to this book - is so enormous that it is only possible to refer to a small fraction of it. Reference to testing on animals *has* been made, though almost exclusively *human viruses* have been discussed in the individual ingredient sections of the book. What is provided in the 55 Supplementary Research Dossiers online represents only a tip of the iceberg in terms of research findings and discussions relevant to the proposal of an 'anti-viral diet'. Additional materials are being added to those research pages regularly in order to keep up-to-date with advances in multiple areas of scientific investigation. Full thanks and appreciation are extended to all of the scientific researchers (including theoretical scientists) whose work has contributed to the composition of this book. At the same time, I wish to emphasize that my acknowledgements do not in any way suggest that any of the scientists whose research is referred to here endorse the current diet. This proposal for an anti-viral diet is a tentative one based on my own understanding of a body of scientific evidence - and for this initial proposition I take full responsibility.

08.08.2020

AVD

the anti-viral diet

BASED ON THE RESULTS OF RECENT
SCIENTIFIC AND MEDICAL RESEARCH

There are in fact two things:
Science and Opinion.
The former begets Knowledge,
the latter Ignorance.

HIPPOCRATES

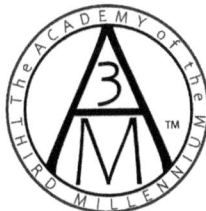

PART 1
A NEW DIET

A NEW DIET

1. ANTI-VIRAL DIET

WHAT IS AN 'ANTI-VIRAL DIET'? - That is perhaps the very first question in need of an immediate answer.

- An 'Anti-Viral Diet' is a diet whose primary purpose is to counteract viral threats and to optimize the ability of our immune systems to fight off both viruses and viral diseases. This volume wishes to present you with a preliminary proposal for an *anti-viral diet*, one that attempts to achieve those aims.

However, no originality is claimed for this idea as there is a significant community of scientists for whom it is common place knowledge that the diets we eat contribute to our ability to fight off - or not - the viruses and diseases in our bodies. What I am attempting to do here is clarify this idea and what might be the bases for believing it is a worthwhile project.

As we live in the presence of the humanly dangerous SARS-CoV-2 virus at this time, I shall endeavour where appropriate to make my comments in the light of this situation and with reference to authorities whose comments are relevant.

On 13th February 2020 - before the World Health Organization had even published any advice on mass gatherings, personal protective equipment or quarantine measures - two Chinese scientists had published an article named 'Potential Interventions for Novel Coronavirus in China: A Systematic Review' in the Journal of Medical Virology. It was, indeed, a solid and systematic piece of work which provided a bird's eye view of what has been learnt in terms of successful treatments for the two previous Coronavirus dangers - SARS and MERS. It covered the use of immuno-enhancers, protease inhibitors, antivirals and other bio-effective compounds, all the while including naturally occurring nutrients within the scope of the study. Pharmaceuticals, dietary ingredients and traditional medicine were all given fair hearing in a fully scientific way. In their preliminary review of the situation, Lei Zhang and Yunhui Liu are confident to assert that general treatments for the Novel Coronavirus – which include nutritional components such as vitamins, minerals *et alia* – are of relevance:

"*We have found that the general treatments are very important to enhance host immune response against RNA viral infection. The immune response has often been shown to be weakened by inadequate nutrition in many model systems as well as in human studies.*"

Indeed, one of their recommendations is that "*the nutritional status of each infected patient should be evaluated before the administration of general treatment*", for this is perhaps the only real way that we will be able to <u>know</u> to what degree nutrituional status may relate to disease progression.

I certainly don't find that a startling conclusion. For we have known for many years that general health is impacted by the balance (often *imbalance*) of nutrients that our bodies receive from the food that we eat. Knowledge that food we eat has an impact on how healthy we are, goes back to the Greeks and beyond: "*Let food be thy medicine and let medicine be thy food*" – those oft-quoted words by Hippocrates, founder of the discipline of medicine itself – are not empty sophistry but appear to have been corroborated by two and a half millennia of scientific research since his day.

In terms of micronutrients – such as vitamins, minerals and other chemicals found in food – two articles published in 'BMJ Nutrition, Prevention & Health' this year properly emphasize the impact that a lack of nutrients can have on our ability to fight off illness – because of how their absence affects our immune system. In the article 'Dietary Micronutrients in the wake of COVID-19', a group of six scientists writes that:

"Existing micronutrient deficiencies, even if only a single micronutrient, can impair immune function and increase susceptibility to infectious disease. Certain population groups are more likely to have micronutrient deficiencies, while certain disease pathologies and treatment practices also exacerbate risk, meaning these groups tend to suffer increased morbidity and mortality from infectious diseases. Optimisation of overall nutritional status, including micronutrients, can be effective in reducing incidence of infectious disease ".

These remarks accentuate the value of ensuring that at least *all known micronutrients* necessary to our body's optimal functioning, be not in short supply. The authors are wholeheartedly reiterating some key findings of Nutritional Science - that the correct levels of body nutrients will contribute to a positive state of health (and likely also lead to a reduction in the occurrence of illness). An article published one month earlier - in May of 2020 - directly emphasizes the value that optimum nutrition can have in the face of illnesses caused by SARS-CoV-2. In 'COVID-19: Is there a Role for Immunonutrition', Emma Derbyshire and Joanne Delange state that:

"Within the nutrition sector a promising body of evidence studying inter-relationships between certain nutrients and immune competence already exists. This could potentially be an important player in helping the body to deal with the coronavirus, especially among elders. Evidence for vitamins C, D and zinc and their roles in preventing pneumonia and respiratory infections (vitamins C and D) and reinforcing immunity (zinc) appears to look particularly promising. Ongoing research within this important field is urgently needed."

If you have already reviewed the contents of **Part 2** of this volume, you may have noticed that the first three sections deal with the inclusion of vitamins, minerals and other vital micro-nutrients in the 'anti-viral diet'. In fact, those groups of ingredients account for a third of the dietary constituents in this book. However, it is clear from the past fifty years of extensive researching into natural agents, that it is not only the well-known micronutrients (such as vitamins, minerals and oils) that have an impact on our ability to deter viruses and disease. Other key ingredients – for example, certain flavonoids, polysaccharides and sesquiterpene lactones found in plants – have proven to be particularly effective in inhibiting viruses through multiple widely different mechanisms of action.

Phytochemicals – chemicals occurring in our natural environment (in plants, foods *etc.*) – have been considered for some decades to be promising avenues for the discovery of new treatment options, as also for the molecular basis of new pharmaceuticals. In an article entitled 'Phytotherapic Compounds against Coronaviruses: Possible Streams for Future Research' – published in April 2020 in Phytotherapy Research – the group of six researchers come to the firm conclusion that:

"phytotherapy research can help to explore potentially useful remedies against coronaviruses, and further investigations are recommended to identify and test all possible targets. Globally, herbs with some preliminary evidence of antiviral activity against coronaviruses, along with phytotherapic remedies with immune stimulant properties, appear as good candidates for additional studies on the topic."

This peer-reviewed article distinguishes between two positive approaches that may be derived from further research into chemicals from nature: *firstly*, herbal remedies with a potentially preventive effect – mainly acting through a general boost of the immune system; and *secondly*, herbal remedies with a potentially therapeutic effect – acting through different mechanisms on viral penetration and replication. Proposals like these, made only a matter of months ago, are neither novel in content nor limited to the scientists who work in the disciplines of plant chemistry, food science or nutrition.

Most notably, one article appeared in the Journal of Applied Microbiology back in 2003 entitled 'Novel Antiviral Agents: A Medicinal Plant Perspective'. Recognizing already then the chasm that exists between laboratory research and the practical application of what is being discovered about phytochemicals, scientists S.A. Jassim and M.A. Naji remark:

"Methods are needed to link antiviral efficacy/potency- and laboratory-based research. Nevertheless, the relative success achieved recently using medicinal plant/herb ex- tracts of various species that are capable of acting therapeu- tically in various viral infections has raised optimism about the future of phyto-antiviral agents. As this review illustrates, there are innumerable potentially useful medicinal plants and herbs waiting to be evaluated and exploited for therapeutic appli- cations against genetically and functionally diverse viruses families."

The authors could hardly be more open-minded about the potential for herbal medicinal plant extracts. They go on to name the *Retroviridae*, *Hepadnaviridae* and *Herpesviri- dae* as examples of disease families against which phyto- chemicals may be used, though they could just as soon have named the *Coronaviridae* also - from which SARS-CoV-2 comes. What reason would there be to suppose that medici- nal plants could not be an option to investigate in relation to that virus as well? Writing over seventeen years ago, S.A. Jas- sim and M.A. Naji observe - in what is a truly wide-ranging review of natural anti-virals: *"Many traditional medicinal plants and herbs were reported to have strong antiviral activity"*, making the further conclusion that:

"In view of the signification [sic.] number of plant ex- tracts that have yielded positive results it seems reasonable to conclude that there are probably numerous kinds of anti- viral agents in these materials."

05

2. <u>THE EVIDENCE</u>

ON THE ONE HAND, it is no surprise to find that those working in the area of 'Alternative Medicine' – as it is very often called – should be excited about the results of some of the research that has been emerging in the past few decades, even be optimistic about the impact that this might have on the current Coronavirus. Writing in the Journal of Traditional and Complementary Medicine in July of 2020, Suraphan Panyod, Chi-Tang Ho and Lee-Yan Sheen give a positive assessment from the traditional viewpoint in their paper 'Dietary Therapy and Herbal Medicine for COVID-19 Prevention' stating that:

"The volume of existing reports is irrefutable evidence that foods and herbs possess a potential antiviral ability against SARS-CoV-2 and can prevent COVID-19. Foods and herbs could be used as dietary or complementary therapy to prevent infection and strengthen immunity."

However, as Alternative Medicine is so often frowned upon by the establishment – which is unfair, in my opinion – it might take the voice of more *serious scientists* in order for the sceptical among us to be convinced of the potential for natural or dietary measures against SARS-CoV-2 and other viruses. An article called 'Natural Products' Role against COVID-19' – published in the journal of the Royal Society of Chemistry (RSC Advances) in June of this year – seems to make similar points to the above article, only using quite a different vocabulary. Ananda da Silva Antonio, Larissa Silveira Moreira Wiedemann and Valdir Florêncio Veiga-Junior write that:

"Bioactivities of natural products have been widely applied in pharmaceutical industry and ethnobotany, such as inflammation, cancer, oxidative process and viral infections. Several antiviral bioproducts have already been described by the activity against Dengue virus, Coronavirus, Enterovirus,

Hepatitis B, Influenza virus and HIV. Thus, bioproducts could be friends in the fight against SARS-CoV-2, through enabling the development of specific chemotherapies to COVID-19. In this paper, we provide insights on the potential of bioproducts in face of this new threat."

Though the Royal Society of Chemistry article specifically mentions 'chemotherapies' being made possible by application of the bioactivities of natural processes, the *dietary application* of bioproducts is certainly not excluded by those authors. Turning back to the article from the Journal of Traditional and Complementary Medicine, I am in agreement with their conclusions – which accord with what I myself have learnt about the past century and a half of scientific research, which revealed many potencies of food and phytochemicals:

"Current literature provides obvious evidence supporting dietary therapy and herbal medicine as potential effective antivirals against SARS-CoV-2 and as preventive agents against COVID-19. Thus, dietary therapy and herbal medicine could be a complementary preventive therapy for COVID-19."

One point that I would like to emphasize, in terms of the current proposal for an anti-viral diet, is that this is not a specifically vegetarian diet as I have not excluded nutrients or chemicals on the grounds that they are most readily available from meat and not plant sources – Iron and L-Carnitine, for example. Both carnivores and herbivores can consume an anti-viral diet, though the ingredients will differ to a degree. Therefore I would not like vegetarians to conclude that I am opposed to their cause – those who, for example, believe that no animals should be killed for human consumption – just as I would not like meat-eaters to infer that this is a vegetarian diet simply because all fifty-two ingredients can be found *in* or *as* plant sources. Though my role is not that of the scientist,

I have tried my best to assess the value of research data that I have referred to, in the most objective way possible. Like a scientist, I do believe that no options should be ignored unless they are shut down by a complete lack of evidence in their favour – or because the facts we have uncovered actually contradict the possibility of a hypothesis having any validity.

Regarding phytochemicals – those food chemicals *derived from plants alone* – I would like to make just a few comments in relation to their importance in the world of medicine. On a conservative estimate, over 70% of medications have their basis in plants. In fact, when you include both medicines which *are derived from plant extracts* and medicines whose chemical structures *are modelled on plant molecules*, then the percentage of medications that originate from nature in one way or another is closer to 85%. Already back in 2007 it was being confirmed in the *Journal of Natural Products* that 70% of medicines introduced into the USA alone have been derived from natural sources – thus a phytochemical basis.

When you expand your view to a wider perspective on our planet, it is worth bearing in mind that the World Health Organization estimates that at least 80% of the world's population rely on traditional medicine of some kind or another – and not on modern pharmaceuticals. It is, of course, very difficult to arrive at truly accurate statistics on such a large scale, but it does appear that several billion people on earth are dependent for their health upon products derived from nature – and not on chemicals synthesized within a laboratory. There are now dozens of journals, published all year round, which report the significant findings from vast domains of plant research being undertaken globally. However, as plant-based medicinal research is such a vast and productive area of scientific investigation, you will find articles reporting results from phytochemical research across all of the major medical and scientific journals also, including Nature, The Lancet, Science, The BMJ, Cell, JAMA and PLoS One - to mention just a few.

In writing the current work, I have found that the majority of research support for the conclusions I have arrived at actually derive from mainstream medical and scientific periodicals - not predominantly from independent journals. Fifty years ago it would have been impossible to refer to such rich sources of research in the areas of plant chemistry and human nutrition, however as ideas of natural antivirals and immuno-nutrition have gradually become mainstream, the research being conducted has grown in every direction and the quantity of data available to draw from now is overwhelming.

Nonetheless, in spite of the high estimation in which natural chemicals are held - both by research communities and the pharmaceutical industry - a peculiar scepticism still persists (even in recent years) around the ability of plants and other food items to be able to prevent, treat or cure medical conditions. When one reflects on the fact that our entire organisms are created from the various manners of sustenance we have taken into our bodies since even before we were born, why should it be so unbelievable that food - *which has formed us* - could have such positive and negative effects on our health? That the nature of food we eat affects our physical well-being in many ways - that hardly seems to be a spectacular conclusion of any kind - on the contrary, mundane.

It has long been a proverb in Germany that *"Man ist was man ißt"* - which in English simply translates as: "You are what you eat". I believe that this is the truth which quietly lies at the core of most every kind of diet. For if the creator of a diet did not believe that altering the intake and nature of food being consumed caused the body to change - then why ever would they have any belief in a diet being beneficial at all?

The global market for the pharmaceutical industry exceeded $1.2 trillion in 2019 - a market that appears to be growing by roughly $100 billion *every year*. When considering the possibility that the right kind of diet might actually be capable of neutralizing viruses and enabling people to overcome both viral and bacterial illnesses more easily – it is hard to ignore the potential impact that this would have on the drug industry. For if people became less reliant on medication – even to a small extent – that would all the same have a cataclysmic impact on the income of the trade in pharmaceuticals. In fact, even if only a small percentage of people acquired a better state of health and better protection from pathogens and illnesses due to following healthier diets, due to the market value that even a small percentage of customers signifies, *this alone* would have a noticeable effect on companies in that sector. Simply massive sums are expended on pharmaceutical products annually, so if an anti-viral diet did become a proven actuality and impact general health, many of the drugs companies would have to reconsider their revenue channels – though *that* is of little concern to most citizens.

What a dream it would be – for so many people of slender means and limited resources – if they were no longer in need of paying large amounts of money just to stay healthy. What an ideal situation it would be if, by following a specific diet, it were possible for us to fight off the many bacteria, viruses and illnesses that attack our bodies on a daily basis. Although much clinical evidence still remains to be gathered, I believe that such a diet is in reach. Before we take a moment to reflect on the current situation – and how such a diet might positively impact this coronaviral scenario – I would like to say a few words about the idea of following a diet, in general.

Even though Merriam-Webster's current English Dictionary entry defines 'Diet' – in one sense only – as "*a regimen of eating and drinking sparingly so as to reduce one's weight*", this is only the fourth and last definition of the word provided, not the central meaning given. In everyday life, however, a 'Diet' **is** most readily understood as referring to a weight-loss program of some kind. In fact that is no surprise, because as far as diets of this type are concerned, more than one thousand different diets for the purpose of 'slimming' have

10

been created in just the past one hundred years. Obesity, for certain, has become a crucial issue of our time. A shocking statistic that has changed little during the past decade, is that on average one third of the population of the U.S.A and U.K. are either obese or overweight. However, even though the issue of how excess fat affects immunity will be addressed in another place, the diet presented here is not a new type of weight-loss program. What is set forth in **AVD** - in terms of a 'Diet' - falls most closely in line with Merriam-Webster's third definition of the word, being *"the kind and amount of food prescribed for a person or animal for a special reason"*.

The 'special reason' for an anti-viral diet is that humans need to be protected from viruses and viral illnesses because other forms of medical prevention and intervention have not yet proved to be successful. I wish to emphasize that I am not referring, in a limited way, to COVID-19. For even once successful cures are proven - in the form of safe anti-viral agents and vaccines, for instance - that will not mean that we are safe from a host of other viruses. The purpose of an anti-viral diet will still be the same, no matter what protection and cures can be provided by pharmaceuticals or other forms of medical treatment - to protect against viruses and viral illnesses.

Research must continue so as to confirm *which natural agents* are capable of disarming *which viruses* - above all, to confirm which natural chemicals can successfully neutralize viruses and viral illnesses in the human body, when ingested. What surprises me, more than anything else, is how in spite of the large amount of evidence that exists in support of an anti-viral diet, none has previously been devised in a scientific way. There have been diets that have moved in the right direction, that is true - especially those which have had as their purpose the optimizing of the human immune system. But in terms of incorporating multiple natural anti-viral agents and immunomodulatory substances - all of which are edible - into an overall diet, I have not found one up to now.

3. <u>A NEW WORLD</u>

AT THE TIME OF WRITING, all nations are still living in peril of the SARS-CoV-2 virus that emerged from China at the end of 2019. Although it is impossible to know for sure, at least half a million deaths are caused annually by influenza viruses alone, yet within just over nine months the SARS-CoV-2 virus is already on track to reaching one million confirmed fatalities through COVID-19 (although some estimate that the numbers may be much larger due to a lack of openness by *some* governments about their national mortality figures). How many million more will die - or whether it will be successfully contained at some point soon - is too hard to say at this moment of crisis. No uniform disease management approaches are being followed by all countries of the world, and that makes it much harder for us to predict what will happen next. Unfortunately, a lack of cooperation between several countries at an earlier stage of this situation has caused COVID-19 to become the largest public health crisis of 2020, even of the past decade - one everyone only wishes would end soon.

It is important to reflect that there are other viral illnesses that are a greater threat to global health and which cause - and have caused - more deaths each year than either Influenza viruses or SARS-CoV-2. Diarrheal illnesses alone account for over two million fatalities between adults and children combined, annually. And 'AIDS' - caused by the Human Immonodeficiency Virus - had already resulted in over 42 million deaths from the 1980s up to 2018. However, even that is less than the 50 million who died of the 'Spanish Flu' from 1918 onwards, and it is absolutely dwarfed by the 300 million deaths which took place from Smallpox in the 20th Century only. Nonetheless, it would be foolish to assume that just those viruses that *have caused* a large trail of bodies are the most dangerous, for there are other viruses - including

Marburg and Ebola - which, although they have been successfully contained during previous outbreaks, can have mortality rates of between 70% to 90%. There are dozens more threatening viruses from which we would need urgent protection if they were to spread, among which Dengue, Zika, Rabies, the Hantavirus and more than it is possible to mention.

However, as this publication is being released at the heart of the COVID-19 pandemic, it is natural that SARS-CoV-2 - more than any other virus - is weighing most heavily on people's minds as they read. It would not be inappropriate, therefore, to spend a moment looking at the impact and development of the current crisis before we look at how an 'anti-viral diet' might be capable of alleviating this situation.

The impact of the Coronavirus SARS-CoV-2 and associated illness COVID-19 have been so massive, that at the height of quarantine measures it was reported by Fox News journalist Chris Ciaccia (5th April 2020) that: "*Coronavirus lockdowns have caused the Earth to effectively stop shaking*". In fact, the American news network was reporting on a piece that had appeared one week earlier in the British scientific journal Nature, where it was reported on March 31st that:

"*efforts to curb the spread of the virus might mean that the planet itself is moving a little less. Researchers who study Earth's movement are reporting a drop in seismic noise — the hum of vibrations in the planet's crust — that could be the result of transport networks and other human activities being shut down*".

The upside was that geologists and other scientists were able to get a better chance than usual to listen to the earthquakes, volcanoes and other geographical occurrences in the world which are ordinarily more difficult to hear because of man-made noise. Thomas Lecocq - a seismologist at the Royal Observatory of Belgium in Brussels - revealed that

the decrease in global movement after the quarantine measures went into place had (quoting Nature) *"caused human-
induced seismic noise to fall by about one-third"*. At no time
previously had sophisticated equipment been able to detect
such a sharp decrease in the sounds created by humankind.
In an oasis of relative calm, it was possible to probe beneath
the waves and under the crust of the earth like never before.

It is amazing to witness how much our planet has alter-
ed over the first nine months of 2020. Where previously the
busy worlds of sport and finance, music and industry, film-
making, travel and education kept this planet buzzing away
each day with a chaotic bustle of activities from first second
to last - for many months there has been silence where before
was nothing but noise, stillness where no-one ever stopped
moving for a moment. Families, businesses, all stayed indoors
or out of action for half the year - even world leaders confin-
ed to their homes. Still at the time of writing - though this may
change by the time you read this - the rates of infection have
been increasing in as many countries as they are decreasing,
while strict measures (including use of face masks, social distancing and quarantine) continue to be enforced by many nations. Nobody knows when things will change - neither exactly
when any vaccine will be administered nor when successful
anti-viral agents will become available. We are living in an
atmosphere of sheer *unpredictability* - that delicate factor
which perhaps affects human nerves, world markets and the
wheel of life more than anything else. The Future is a Blank.

17:43, 30th December 2019 - Dr. Li Winliang of Wuhan
Central Hospital warns some of his medical peers in a post
on Chinese social media site 'WeChat' that a Coronavirus -
similar to the deadly SARS - is making the rounds and urges
them all to take protective measures: *"7 confirmed cases of
SARS were reported* [to hospital] *from Huanan Seafood Market"*, adding later in the day that *"the latest news is, it has*

been confirmed that they are coronavirus infections, but the exact virus strain is being subtyped". However, instead of being thanked and praised for his timely advance warning – before there had been any larger outbreak – Dr. Winliang was swiftly faced with prosecution.

On 3rd January 2020, the doctor was interrogated by police from the Wuhan Public Security Bureau. He was given a stern warning notice that censured him for *"making false comments on the Internet "* and then he was forced to sign a 'letter of admonition' in which he had to promise that he would say no more. – After having returned to work at Wuhan Central Hospital, by January 8th it was apparent that Dr. Linwiang had fallen victim to an infection himself. In contact with one of his patients – whom he suspected of having this coronavirus – he contracted an illness and by 10th January he had developed a fever and a cough. His deterioration was rapid enough: by 12th January he was admitted to the intensive care department, by 1st February he was finally diagnosed with this viral infection – and by 6th February he was dead. His death was first announced by Chinese state media, although this announcement was soon after deleted by them, while Wuhan Central Hospital was not prepared to say more than that:

"In the process of fighting the coronavirus, the eye doctor from our hospital Li Wenliang was unfortunately infected. He is now in critical condition and we are doing our best to rescue him".

However the reality is that he had already died – and from the viral illness that he himself discovered and feared.

His story would not be forgotten, for on 31st January – only one week before his demise – the resilient doctor had shared his tale on the internet. He spoke up about his not having been allowed to speak of what he knew, and he promised that he would rejoin his colleagues at work soon. His post soon went viral and in the wake of Linwiang's death the hashtag #wewantfreedomofspeech gained over two million views and over 5,500 posts within only 5 hours – only to be removed soon thereafter by the Chinese State censors.

The World Health Organization were to post on Twitter [@WHO] that: *"We are saddened by the passing of Dr Li Wenliang"* and *"We all need to celebrate work that he did on #2019nCoV"*. However, by February 2020 the fate of so many of us had already been sealed as the Novel Coronavirus SARS-CoV-2 had been allowed to wander in silence and freedom to all corners of the earth. There are certainly a number of people who have expressed the opinion that it might have been better if WHO were less willing to merely take the Chinese Government at its word. Indeed – still by 14th January 2020 – the World Health Organization were reporting that:

"Preliminary investigations conducted by the Chinese authorities have found no clear evidence of human-to-human transmission of the novel #coronavirus (2019-nCoV) identified in #Wuhan, #China."

Bolstered, perhaps, by the light-hearted approach of WHO, President Donald J. Trump of the United States was happy enough to joke about the Coronavirus just being the Democrat Party's *"New Hoax"*, even going so far as to say – based on no scientific evidence available then – that it would be going away with warmer weather and that, in any case, it was *"totally under control"*.

Nothing could have been any further from the truth, yet it was not only the USA and China who shared the view that this new, infectious virus was of negligible harm. For even Professor Didier Raoult of Marseilles, now widely acclaimed for his repurposing of the malarial drug Hydroxychloroquine as a viable treatment option for COVID-19, originally said of this Coronavirus – after remarking that there are a greater number of scooter deaths in Italy than from the new virus – that:

"Every year there are tens of millions of deaths in the world due to viral respiratory infections. There will be a few hundred more. If you look at the new cases, the rate of new contamination is less than 1% right now; it's very low and it suggests that the epidemic is coming to an end".

Writing in the second half of 2020, any nonchalance from the first half of this year just shows how impossible it is to predict the course of a virus. While MERS and SARS - both more dangerous than SARS-CoV-2 in terms of their mortality rates - were succesfully contained before either of them could become a global catastrophe, viral disease COVID-19 continues to cause thousands of deaths daily with no end in sight.

From where I stand now, I see a World in Panic, our lives still paralysed by Fear. Microscopic virions have indeed managed to conquer the globe and we are behaving just as anxiously as if aliens had landed here. 'War of the Worlds' comes to mind, though ironically *there* it is the aliens who are defeated by bacteria - while *here* it is we who are at the mercy of a virus. It should be clear by now that even though viruses are smaller than the most minuscule of bacteria - and could not be seen until the advent of electron microscopes - they are capable of destroying lives more effectively and systematically than any war. 'Extra terrestrials' they are not, but *brand new terrestrials* they are - for even though the complex encoded particles of the SARS-CoV-2 virus may have evolved from other strains of the 'Corona' family, now they are life forms that are unique in themselves. Correction : *viruses are not actually deemed to be lives in themselves* - for they are incapable of living without the help of other organisms and unable to replicate themselves unless they use an actual lifeform to help them do so. Much like the aliens in 'Invasion of the Body Snatchers' - who use human bodies as 'pods' within which to grow - viruses have to hijack the bodies of plants or animals (including the human species) in order to successfully replicate themselves. Without their hosts, they are helpless.

17

4. CORONAVIRUSES

CORONAVIRUSES ARE NOT NEW. We were to identify the very first of them – in humans – during the Beatles decade, though the identification of coronaviruses in animals had already occurred by the 1930s, when some severe upper respiratory tract infections were diagnosed in chickens. By last year, six coronaviruses in total had been discovered in humans, two of which have proven themselves to be a lethal threat to our species: 'MERS-CoV' and 'SARS-CoV-1'.

The coronaviruses that were first discovered in humans date back over fifty years and were identified in patients with symptoms like those of a common cold. In fact, two coronaviruses that affect humans – named '229E' and 'OC43' – are both responsible for some common colds and do not generally lead to more serious complications, except in those who are compromised by other conditions or infections. Two more of the human coronaviruses are not necessarily lethal in nature, although they are more concerning. Coronavirus 'NL63' was isolated as a unique strain in 2004 and – like the two foregoing viruses – was found to be responsible for chest infections as found in an influenza, in some cases capable of causing Severe Acute Respiratory Syndrome. As for human coronavirus 'HKU1' – discovered in 2005 – this is also more aggressive than both 229E and OC43, causing respiratory infections and being able to bring about pneumonia and bronchiolitis in a number of patients. Considered together, the four coronaviruses mentioned in this paragraph do not pose a deadly threat to humans, while their accompanying illnesses can be treated successfully on the majority of occasions.

However, as is widely known, some coronaviruses are a much greater threat to human life. In 2012, for example, a new type of coronavirus was identified in Saudi Arabia and further afield in the Middle East. It was originally called 'Novel

Coronavirus 2012', although it has since become officially known as 'Middle East Respiratory Syndrome Coronavirus' or simply MERS-CoV. Even though the World Health Organization originally announced a global alert on the 24th of September 2012 - regarding the danger of the illness it causes - by the 28th of that same month they had reassured countries that this virus did not seem to pass easily from human to human. However, cases of human transmission *were recorded* in multiple instances, so it had to be confirmed that it was in fact contagious. What was most perturbing about 'MERS' (in terms of resultant illnesses). was that in spite of there appearing to be low infection rates of the virus between humans - as people were generally infected by animals with the virus - the mortality rate was recorded to be as high as 35%.

Even though most people infected with MERS would develop only moderate symptoms - and there were even those showing no symptoms - many complications could occur, including severe pneumonia (leading to acute respiratory distress syndrome), kidney failure, disseminated intravascular coagulation (where small blood-clots occur throughout the bloodstream) and pericarditis (an inflammation of two layers of tissue surrounding the heart, which can stop it working). Any of the above problems could lead to death and in one review of the cases occurring in Saudi Arabia, it was recorded that over 70% of MERS patients required mechanical ventilation. The MERS-CoV has had three outbreaks - in 2012, 2015 and 2018 - with 27 countries affected, 2494 cases confirmed by WHO and over 858 deaths recorded worldwide in total.

However, it was in fact a whole decade earlier that the closest predecessor to the SARS-CoV-2 virus emerged - a virus originally named SARSr-CoV - but now called SARS-CoV-1, distinguishing it from the present virus. An illness surfaced with flu-like symptoms, one that could include muscle pain, lethargy, cough and sore throat, plus a symptom that was common to all patients - fever above 38 °C (100 °F).

Like MERS, SARS was a spill-over from animal species – but whereas in the former case people appear to have been infected by camels, in the latter case it was identified as first originating from cave-dwelling horseshoe bats from Yunnan (China). Like COVID-19, SARS can lead to shortness of breath and several types of pneumonia, in some cases being fatal. As is known by many people now – due to the present pandemic – the abbreviation S.A.R.S. stands for 'Severe Acute Respiratory Syndrome' as this is one of the main conditions that it causes, which impacts the lungs' ability to function properly.

Thankfully, in spite of the initial delay in sharing information about the virus by the Chinese, the SARS outbreak of 2002-2003 was successfully contained and the total number of cases amounted to 8096, with 774 deaths occurring in all. The very last recorded case appears to have taken place in 2004, no other instances of SARS being reported since then.

Like the current virus, the spread of SARS-CoV-1 is able to be prevented by numerous practical means – ones that can be effective with a great many viruses: regular hand-washing with soap and water (or alcohol-based hand sanitizer), disinfection of any objects or surfaces that the virus might survive on, plus making people stay at home who might be infected – whether exhibiting illness or not. In fact, there is currently no cure either for SARS or the aforementioned MERS illness – no vaccines exist, thus social isolation and quarantine measures are the most successful ways to prevent proliferation of cases.

In one sense, the occurrence of both these coronaviruses so recently had given researchers and governments a 'heads-up' on how to manage the 2020 'Coronademic', for the majority of measures that were effective then can be just just as effective now. Both of the SARS-CoVs, for example, are crucially spread through respiratory droplets in the air, therefore the use of face-masks (and provision in the correct quantity to all key services workers) should have happened immediately and not like some clumsy afterthought – as in the UK.

Where airport screening processes, quarantining and social distancing had all proven to be successful procedures previously, the governments worldwide should have instigated those same systems of action in a coördinated way. Sadly, this has not been the case and it is impossible to calculate the amount of medical, societal and financial damage that has been caused through lack of effective measures being taken by some countries and want of coördination in general. One can only hope that with the realization of how severely early mistakes in containment can let an evil Genii out of the bottle - future contagions may be limited by better management. Soderbergh's 'Contagion' seems to have predicted so many of the mistakes that would be made, one decade ago.

Initially identified by Dr. Lin Winliang, of Wuhan Hospital in December 2019, the current virus was initially called '2019-nCov' before being named 'SARS-CoV-2' by the International Committee on Taxonomy of Viruses on 11th February 2020. Since then, by the time of writing this book COVID-19 - the disease caused by SARS-CoV-2 - is headed towards 30 million cases globally and will soon reach 1 million deaths. The incubation period is relatively long - ranging up to two weeks, or more in some cases - and is most contagious during the first three days. Typical symptoms of COVID-19 are fever, a cough, tiredness and difficulties in breathing - sometimes just shortness of breath. Stomach related symptoms have also been reported in a significant number of patients and loss of sense of smell has been added to the official list of symptoms. As in the case of SARS, more serious instances of the illness include pneumonia and acute respiratory distress syndrome. Like SARS also, the current virus appears to be a spill-over from animals, possibly bats - although the spread first originated from a seafood market in Wuhan. Currently there is no prescribed cure for COVID-19 though there are well over 300 vaccines in development. No clinical trials have been completed and there is no agreement on a safe antiviral agent.

5. <u>SEARCH FOR A CURE</u>

ON JANUARY 29th 2020 The Lancet Journal published an article presenting a description of *"the genomic structure of a seventh human coronavirus that can cause severe pneumonia"* – the SARS-CoV-2 virus. From nine patient samples the 35 scientists managed to document seven complete genome sequences, exhibiting more than 99·98% sequence identity.

From the moment that the genetic (RNA) sequence of SARS-CoV-2 had been shared in the scientific community, researchers and innovators worldwide have had an opportunity to analyse and understand the workings of this 'Novel Coronavirus' and to attempt to find a cure down whatever routes they felt might be most fruitful. Research and investigation has branched out in various directions and it is likely that there will ultimately not be one, but many ways in which to defeat SARS-CoV-2 and concomitant illness COVID-19.

On 11th March 2020, Dr. Tedros Adhanom Ghebreyesus, WHO's Director-General, first announced that COVID-19 could be characterized as a pandemic, stating that:

"WHO has been assessing this outbreak around the clock and we are deeply concerned both by the alarming levels of spread and severity, and by the alarming levels of inaction. We have therefore made the assessment that COVID-19 can be characterized as a pandemic. Pandemic is not a word to use lightly or carelessly. It is a word that, if misused, can cause unreasonable fear, or unjustified acceptance that the fight is over, leading to unnecessary suffering and death."

However, already four weeks earlier – in the Journal of Medical Virology – scientists Lei Zhang and Yunhui Liu had set forth over three dozen potential interventions which might be successful in defeating COVID-19. One of their key suggestions was that since SARS and MERS are so closely related to SARS-CoV-2 (from the same virus family) it would be worthwhile reviewing treatments for *those* illnesses as part of our search for viable treatment options. Already in their 'Introduction' they remark on the familial connection between the three viruses:

"*Recently, a novel flu-like coronavirus (COVID-19) related to the MERS and SARS coronaviruses was found at the end of 2019 in China, and the evidence of human-to-human transmission was confirmed among close contacts. The genome of COVID-19 is a single-stranded positive-sense RNA. The sequence analysis showed that the COVID-19 possessed a typical genome structure of coronavirus and belonged to the cluster of β-coronaviruses including SARS-CoV and MERS-CoV. COVID-19 was more than 82% identical to those of SARS-CoV.*"

The authors are not in disagreement with the generally accepted goal of a vaccine for COVID-19. There are half a dozen different sorts of vaccine possible but there is no space to enumerate those types here. However, the 'Centers for Disease Control and Prevention' summarize the general point as: "*Vaccines help develop immunity by imitating an infection*". In their useful leaflet from July 2018, entitled 'Understanding How Vaccines Work', the CDC explains how vaccines – whether these use all or part of a virus, live *or* inactivated – can stimulate the body's immune system in the correct way so that it learns how to fight off the same virus if exposed to it again:

"*Once the imitation infection goes away, the body is left with a supply of "memory" T-lymphocytes, as well as B-lymphocytes that will remember how to fight that disease in the future.*"

However, in the absence of any developed vaccine at that time, the authors made one very relevant observation from which they derive a valid query: are children less likely to get COVID-19 due to having received vaccines for other RNA viruses (such as Measles) more recently than adults?

"*children are seldom attacked by COVID-19 as well as SARS-CoV. It may be due to the required vaccine program for every child. The RNA-virus vaccines and the adjuvants in vaccine programs may help children escape from the infection. Therefore, the RNA-virus-related vaccines including measles (MeV), polio, Japanese encephalitis virus, influenza virus, and rabies-related vaccines, could be used as the most promising alternative choices to prevent human-to-human transmission through immunizing health care workers and noninfected population as well.*"

They also suggest 'convalescent plasma' as a treatment for critically ill patients as it had been successful in MERS and SARS cases before. The principle is that the blood of a person recovering from a coronavirus contains antibodies that will counteract the virus, even in another person's body:

"*- convalescent plasma had an immunotherapeutic potential for the treatment of MERS-CoV infection. In addition, convalescent plasma from recovered SARS patients had also been reported to be useful clinically for treating other SARS patients. Importantly, the use of convalescent plasma or serum was also suggested by the World Health Organization under Blood Regulators Network when vaccines and antiviral drugs were unavailable for an emerging virus.*"

Otherwise, in addition to the identification of thirty different chemicals that previous research indicates may counteract the virus, Zhang and Liu recommend 'monoclonal antibody therapy' as one of the best forms of passive immunotherapy. - Even at the beginning of 2020 there was no lack of prospective treatment options for COVID-19 - the only thing missing was the clinical data verifying that these interventions can actually be successful for COVID-19 patients in practice.

For anyone interested in the wide range of treatment options that can be considered, this article is one of the best starting points. It takes into account general treatment options as well as more targeted ones. The effect of micronutrients on coronaviruses is covered, the impact of immunoenhancers – such as interferons and intravenous gammaglobulin – and even the possibility of traditional medicinal agents is not ignored.

As far as coronaviral protease inhibitors are concerned – which are able to block replication of the viruses – this article already identified Chloroquine as one of the likely candidates for success, one month before Professor Raoult announced the promising results of his initial trials in Marseille, France.

Antivirals such as Remdesivir and Ribavirin were also on Zhang's and Lui's list of options, though they also included naturally occurring antivirals like Alpha-Lipoic acid and Estradiol. This is in line with the general attitude of the authors of that review – that science should be as open-minded about evaluating natural chemicals as it is with pharmaceutical agents.

The important observation of theirs within that review – quoted earlier – that the dietary intake of patients may be one determining factor in the development of illness, is worth reiterating here: "*The immune response has often been shown to be weakened by inadequate nutrition in many model systems as well as in human studies*", from which they conclude:

"*Therefore, we propose to verify the nutritional status of COVID-19 infected patients before the administration of general treatments.*"

In general, this article from the Journal of Medical Virology points toward micronutrients, natural chemicals and traditional medicinal agents as valid candidates for anti-viral and immuno-enhancing treatment options for COVID-19.

A NOTE ON IMMUNITY

MY MAIN CONCERN in trying to condense an anti-viral diet into a 200-page paperback, is that there is no way that the intricacies of how viruses and the immune system interact with each other can be discussed. However, a few words on the topic of 'Immunity' and the way in which the body copes with attacks on it in general, may be of benefit to some readers.

The first thing to understand is that the body's immune system has the ability to identify the difference between the SELF and the NON-SELF. When a foreign object of some kind enters our own bodies, the immune system recognizes that it is a NON-SELF molecule, and that something needs to be done about it. Foreign objects that may be of harm to the human body are called 'Pathogens' and are of various types. Bacteria, Viruses and Fungi are three forms of pathogen. The difference between <u>bacteria</u> and <u>viruses</u> is that the former are officially a life form - consisting of a biological cell with a simple internal structure but no nucleus - while the latter are not actually "*alive*". Viruses, invisible to traditional microscopes, can only replicate themselves within the cells of a living organism - and for that reason do not satisfy all criteria of 'Life'.

As most textbooks on biology will teach you, there are two types of immunity. When the human body detects that a pathogen has breached its surface - for example, the dirt in a grazed knee - then an instant and automatic reaction happens in which the immune system sends in a 'soldier level' of white blood cells and chemical agents to deal with the disaster. Strange feelings may occur in your wound, different liquids appearing, blood clotting and skin perhaps changing colour. This kind of immediate response - that occurs in all animals - is called 'Innate Immunity' and is described as being 'non-specific' in the way it reacts to pathogens, because it follows the same script every time. Sometimes this type of immune reaction can become a negative occurrence because of the

26

severity of the human body's response. The 'Cytokine Storms' of COVID-19 actually result from a dangerous over-reaction of the human immune system – and as is well known, such crisis situations can become so severe that they lead to death.

The more intriguing side of the immune system – only to be found in jawed vertebrates – is called 'Acquired Immunity'. This is because it refers to the ability of the body to acquire knowledge about the nature of specific pathogens and how it can successfully deal with them. Whereas the 'Innate' type of immunity is like an instant reaction, in the case of 'Acquired' immunity there is a lag time between being subjected to a pathogen and mounting a response. This is because the body is using complex mechanisms within the hierarchy of white blood cells (plus other chemical agents in the blood) so as to identify the pathogen in question – and if a previous attack has been fended off successfully, then the same type of campaign can be mounted again. Where Innate Immunity fails, Acquired Immunity will step in and try to solve the problem instead. 'Immunological Memory' refers to that element of the immune system which remembers what worked – using that memory so as to effect a maximal response to the pathogen. If a person *has recovered* from a viral infection, it is possible that their body will have learnt how to fight off the same viral threat in future, more easily (though this is not *always* true). As for immunizations, these are a clever instance of pre-infecting a person with a certain virus so that their body will be capable of mounting an intelligent response if re-exposed to that virus.

One point I would like to raise here, is that one of the key requirements of a well-functioning immune system is that it communicates within itself effectively. When that happens, there is a greater likelihood that the body will mount the response that is most appropriate to overcoming the pathogenic threat. Over-reactions and insufficient reactions by the immune system occur when there are communication problems.

6. <u>BASED UPON TRUTH</u>

SCIENCE IS BASED UPON TRUTH. The raw data of what happens in reality are the substance upon which the conclusions of science (and medicine) are based. That is why relying on the results of scientific and medical research appears to me to be the only acceptable basis for any potential anti-viral diet. Old wives' tales, rumours of magical ingredients and the opinions of the press and social media - these, on the other hand, can only lead towards chaos, contradiction and confusion.

Based on a review of articles published by over five thousand authors across the disciplines of microbiology, medicine, virology, nutrition, biogenetics, phytochemistry and the study of infectious diseases - I have discovered what I deem to be significant evidence supportive of such an anti-viral diet. American and British researchers as much as those working in China and India, research into microbiology and pathogenics as much as that in organic chemistry and food science - the corroboration for **AVD** derives from multifarious disciplines and arises from the work of different types of scientists.

Science needs to be objective and ready to approach any proposed theory in terms of experimention and results. - Evidence that nutrition makes a difference to our immune system, that natural antiviral agents exist, as well as that there are dietary ingredients that inhibit the replication of viruses through numerous biochemical mechanisms - all this is on the record. After studying the findings from a large body of articles and monographs, I became convinced that the existing evidence of science does support the proposition of an anti-viral diet. I realize, however, that my own attempt is only a preliminary one, and the inclusion or exclusion of different dietary elements (than those presented in this volume) may occur over time. As the results of scientific research - taking place now and over the coming years - will develop and transform our knowledge of the immune system and viruses, it is inevitable that the diet itself will change. A considerable amount of work also needs to be done in terms of reviewing the most relevant evidence in corroboration of this preliminary anti-viral diet.

At this moment in time, however, as the project of an anti-viral diet may still be considered something quite novel and not yet validated by science, I think it may be best if we hear from a few more voices in the scientific community regarding the general ideas behind such a different kind of diet.

As far as a very general question is concerned - *whether diet can affect infectivity* (and also specifically in regards to infectivity by SARS-CoV-2) - an article published at the end of May 2020 in Clinical & Translational Allergy appears to confirm this in the affirmative. Regarding the impact of what we eat on the immune system, and viral vulnerability, the paper 'Is Diet Partly Responsible for Differences in COVID-19 Death Rates between and within Countries?' asserts that:

"Nutrition may therefore play a role in the immune defense against COVID-19 and may explain some of the differences seen in COVID-19 across Europe. It will be needed to test dietary differences between low and high-rate countries. Foods with potent antioxidant or anti ACE activity — like uncooked or fermented cabbage — are largely consumed in low-death rate European countries, Korea and Taiwan, and might be considered in the low prevalence of deaths."

Although the above comment is quite general in nature, not taking into account alternative parameters that could be responsible for the difference in mortality rates across different countries - the evidence and analysis exists if one does wish to drill down to more detailed specifics; for instance, regarding the relationship between fermented food and mortality. In that case, one need only turn to a more targeted article like

'Association between Consumption of Fermented Vegetables and COVID-19 Mortality at a Country Level in Europe' (medRxiv) published in July this year, where it is stated more precisely:

"Mortality counts were analyzed with quasi-Poisson regression models - with log of population as an offset - to model the death rate while accounting for over-dispersion. Results: Of all the variables considered, including confounders, only fermented vegetables reached statistical significance with the COVID-19 death rate per country. For each g/day increase in the average national consumption of fermented vegetables, the mortality risk for COVID-19 decreased by 35.4% (95% CI: 11.4%, 35.5%)."

Even though sciences like nutrition, phytotherapy, biogenetics and immunology are relatively new, genuine mountain-ranges of data and findings are already in existence. Whatever aspect of the Food-Health relationship one wishes to explore, research is already out there. While the above paper gets us further into details about the relationship between fermented food consumption and incidence of death, it is just as easy to find more exact information about how nutrition affects the immune system. For example, this review article from the Diabetology & Metabolic Syndrome journal - entitled 'Enhancing Immunity in Viral Infections, with Special Emphasis on COVID-19' - provides more accurate analysis:

"As evident from the studies described above, micronutrient deficiency suppresses immune functions by affecting the T-cell-mediated immune response and adaptive antibody response, and leads to dysregulation of the balanced host response. Selected vitamins and trace elements support immune function by strengthening epithelial barriers and cellular and humoral immune responses. Supplementations with various combinations of trace-elements and vitamins have shown beneficial effects on the antiviral immune response."

As the anti-viral effect of several dietary elements derives from their immunomodulatory properties, it is pertinent that the positive impact ingredients can have on the immune system has been widely recognized in the scientific literature. One need only read a paper like Prof. Philip Calder's 'Feeding the Immune System' (with over 150 highly relevant references) so as to appreciate this. From the abstract of this paper alone - appearing in the Proceedings of the Nutrition Society in 2013 - it is clear *how much* science has to teach us about the intimate relations between food and the immune system:

> "*Practically all forms of immunity are affected by protein-energy malnutrition, but non-specific defences and cell-mediated immunity are most severely affected. Micronutrient deficiencies impair immune function. Here, vitamins A, D and E, and Zn, Fe and Se are discussed. The gut-associated lymphoid tissue is especially important in health and well-being because of its close proximity to a large and diverse population of organisms in the gastrointestinal tract and its exposure to food constituents. Certain probiotic bacteria which modify the gut microbiota enhance immune function in laboratory animals and may do so in human subjects.*"

Joanne Delange and Emma Derbyshire sum up this view succinctly - in their previously cited article 'COVID-19: Is there a Role for Immunonutrition' - when they say that: "*Balanced nutrition which can help in maintaining immunity is essential for prevention and management of viral infections.*"

In terms of the ingredients that are included in **AVD**, it is true that the majority of them do have a direct or indirect impact on the functioning of the immune system. However, there are also dietary elements whose main benefit is not in enhancing immune response but rather in disarming viruses according to various biochemical mechanisms. Obviously, it was vital to this diet that there be sufficient evidence to prove that some ingredients included actually exert those effects. Regarding a few of the traditional constituents included in this diet – some of which have a history of being used in Chinese Medicine – an article from the journal Nutrients, entitled 'The Antiviral, Anti-Inflammatory Effects of Natural Medicinal Herbs and Mushrooms and SARS-CoV-2 Infection', tells us:

"The extracts described in this review have been proven to possess great antiviral activities, with a general consensus of low toxicity. In addition, compared to commercial pharmaceuticals, such medicinal herbs are readily available and much cheaper. With the current pandemic, many scientists have rushed to the development of a potential vaccine and therapeutic agent that is effective against COVID-19; however, herbal agents should not be overlooked."

Elsewhere, in peer-reviewed research journal Frontiers in Medicine, the article 'Plants Metabolites: Possibility of Natural Therapeutics Against the COVID-19 Pandemic' comes to similar conclusions based on its inquiries, summing up that:

"Our investigation revealed that the proposed plant metabolites can serve as potential anti-SARS-CoV-2 lead molecules for further optimization and drug development processes to combat COVID-19 and future pandemics caused by viruses. This review will stimulate further analysis by the scientific community and boost antiviral plant-based research."

One particular avenue of value in the development of an anti-viral diet – which could not have been relied on before *as the means did not exist* – is the use of computational analysis of molecular interactions in order to predict which chemicals (whether natural or synthetic) are likely to 'inhibit' a virus by docking with it in a competitive way. One particular study of this kind, making use of advanced molecular docking simulation software, tested a number of pharmaceutical (control) compounds at the same time as exploring a large number of natural agents. The article 'An Investigation into the Identification of Potential Inhibitors of SARS-CoV-2 Main Protease using Molecular Docking Study' - published in the Journal of Bio-molecular Structure and Dynamics in May 2020 - shares findings from that research, which are truly significant:

"Here, in this study, we have utilized a blind molecular docking approach to identify the possible inhibitors of the SARS-CoV-2 main protease, by screening a total of 33 molecules which includes natural products, anti-virals, anti-fungals, anti-nematodes and anti-protozoals. All the studied molecules could bind to the active site of the SARS-CoV-2 protease (PDB: 6Y84), out of which rutin (a natural compound) has the highest inhibitor efficiency among the 33 molecules studied, followed by ritonavir (control drug), emetine (anti-protozoal), hesperidin (a natural compound), lopinavir (control drug) and indinavir (anti-viral drug)."

Another 'in silico' study, published in Acta Pharmaceutica Sinica B, that same month, provided equally important results. In the 'Analysis of Therapeutic Targets for SARS-CoV-2 and Discovery of Potential Drugs by Computational Methods', the thirteen scientists on that investigation concluded:

"The natural products, such as flavanoids like neohesperidin, hesperidin, baicalin, kaempferol 3-O-rutinoside and rutin from different sources, andrographolide, neoandrographolide and 14-deoxy-11,12-didehydroandrographolide from A. paniculata, and a series of xanthones from the plants of Swertia genus, with anti-virus, anti-bacteria and anti-inflammation activity could effectively interact with these targets of SARS-CoV-2. Therefore, the herbal medicines containing these compounds as major components might be meaningful for the treatment of SARS-CoV-2 infections."

In terms of the natural, edible and herbal elements in the current diet, only those for which sufficient evidence exists have been included here. In each case, at least a dozen scientific research papers corroborate their position in this diet, in some cases twice as many. As for the issue of COVID-19, over 80% of the ingredients in **AVD** have evidence in support of their beneficial effect against SARS-CoV-2 and its illness. I mention that at this point as I fully realize that a number of-readers may have turned to this volume in search of a therapeutic option for COVID-19. There are two points which I wish to emphasize regarding that: *Firstly*, no guarantees are made by this anti-viral diet in any way whatsoever. All that is asserted here is that the inclusion of a larger number of natural anti-viral agents in one's diet will *likely decrease the probability of one contracting some viral illnesses.* - *Secondly*, although this edition does place a particular focus on anti-viral agents effective against SARS-CoV-2 and COVID-19, the aim of this book has not been to devise a diet specific to that virus and illness, but to arrive at a preliminary anti-viral diet that may offer a level of dietary protection against viruses in general.

In terms of considering the use of natural ingredients in order to overcome the presently challenging scenario, I find the June article from the Royal Society of Chemistry's journal RSC Advances is most refreshng and energizing in its attitude to 'Natural products' role against COVID-19'. There, the three authors Ananda da Silva Antonio, Larissa Silveira Moreira Wiedemann and Valdir Florêncio Veiga-Junior write that:

"*In the face of this great global challenge, we are striving for a COVID-19 treatment that can be quickly produced and easily distributed. Natural products could provide an answer to this dilemma, as they often have low toxicity and are used in the pharmaceutical industry for their bioactivity, including antiviral.*"

- For scientists, words of great optimism.

7. <u>PERSONAL CHOICE</u>

A DIET IS A PERSONAL CHOICE. What we eat and drink and when and how – *that* is not a matter of science or evidence. Eating meals at one or more times of the day, having various types of refreshment – and perhaps some snacks too – those are personal decisions, choices that we make on a daily basis.

All that I have described in the preceding sections – and attempted to support with some preliminary observations – is the *idea of an anti-viral diet in general*. It is, in the first place an <u>idea</u>. The question is whether this can go from being a mere concept to being a diet that people follow in reality. Obviously, the proposition of being able to protect oneself from viruses and viral threats, through adopting a diet alone – is a very attractive one. However, even once the most effective balance of anti-viral dietary ingredients has been identified, there will still be a distance to go in order to customize that base diet for the many background health conditions that people have – some of which do restrict ingredient choices.

The purpose of the remainder of this publication is to introduce you to the 52 dietary ingredients which – especially used in combination – may be able to protect against a large variety of viruses, though more clinical trial data is still needed regarding the majority of them. Science will not be satisfied until something is *proven*, and that is how it should be. Science is here to protect us from rumours and superstition – like Law, it is only interested in facts and evidence, the rest immaterial.

After **Part 2** of this publication has presented you with the components of this first Anti-Viral Diet – providing you with the research basis of their anti-viral and immunomodulatory properties – **Part 3** will move on to the stage of helping you to design your own daily diet, including those ingredients.

Whether you actually decide to try out this diet is, I realize, dependent on a number of different factors which will vary from person to person: how satisfied you are with the scientific evidence existing now, whether you feel safe about the balance of benefit-to-risk - and also, I guess, what your gut-feelings are about changing what you eat every day.

We've considered the evidence issues briefly in a couple of the previous sections, though I think you will only really be able to make your mind up on the data relating to each of the ingredients once you have progressed to **Part 2** of **AVD**.

It is understandable - and advisable, I believe - when considering a decision which will have a personal and medical impact in one's life, that you have to balance the benefits and risks. What will be the risks that you expose yourself to if you do not take additional steps to protect yourself from viral dangers? What are the benefits that could come from ingesting the anti-viral agents if their efficacy proved successful for you? Are there potential dietary risks that need to be carefully weighed up due to any condition you have? What about the benefits improving your diet could have on your family life?

To balance these factors - and others - is a natural and essential part of deciding whether to follow this diet. In the end, all any person can do is to make decisions based upon what they know and how they feel about it all - a combination of balancing up priorities and evaluating probabilities.

At the end of the day, even when you take prescribed medication, your doctor cannot **know** - in advance of your taking it - whether a certain medicine will be effective or not. You both have to wait and see what the results will be.

I find it perfectly understandable that some people will be dubious of a diet which, even though its claims are supported or indicated by scientific evidence has not yet been proven in clinical trials. Test-tube experiments, animal trials and molecular simulations - all of these are of great value in arriving at knowledge of dietary ingredients, but naturally nothing could ever be of more value than full observation and documenting of the actual effects that ingestion of an ingredient has on a person's proneness to viruses and their levels of immunity. For those who wish to wait while more trials are undertaken and as more statistics are gathered - before venturing upon what is an 'experimental diet' - I fully understand.

However, I do also appreciate that there are many people who - either due to lack of resources, money or government- provided healthcare - are in need of an alternative option when it comes to overcoming the present Coronavirus and other viruses that may be affecting their countries. Starting with changes in diet that might increase their levels of immunity and decrease how vulnerable people are to viruses, could be a most practical and affordable way to proceed.

The current Coronavirus has not yet decreased in the threat it poses to society. The virus is no less contagious and dangerous now - there is no room for complacency in terms of containment measures that countries have initiated: social distancing, quarantining, use of personal protective equipment and optimized hygiene, to name a few. Every nation, considering the easing of such restrictions, has good reason to worry whether in doing so there will result an increase of the viral spread - as a consequence lose months of ground on whatever progress has been made countering the illness.

Although, as author of **AVD**, I do follow this diet myself and have not succumbed to any illness - bacterial or viral - since doing so, I do not mention this fact as any form of conclusive evidence or proof that the diet 'works in reality' but just in order to make it plain that "*I practice what I preach*".

What **Part 3** has offered me, more than this opening essay or the presentation of ingredients, is an opportunity to chat with you in detail about how one can manage to incorporate the different elements of **AVD** into one's own life - even when you only have a limited time to think about food choices.

Hippocrates - in the body of the Oath which is sworn by all who join the medical profession - stresses the importance a doctor has in managing their patient's diet properly:

"I will use those dietary regimens which will benefit my patients according to my greatest ability and judgment."

Personally, I think that there is a silent knowledge, deep within the micro-substance of our body's very cells, that what we eat makes a fundamental difference to what we are, including whether we become ill frequently or remain healthy. I think that someone eating excess amounts of unhealthy fat has a 'gut-feeling' that it isn't good for them, even while they continue with this harmful behaviour. I equally believe that when another person is eating some raw fruit and vegetables - as a part of their diet - they may have an intuitive sense that there is something right about this. Perhaps I am saying this based on my own personal perspective, for there have been a number of occasions when I *knew* that food was not doing me any good - and subsequently fell ill - as well as an equal number of times when I knew precisely what to eat in order to make my stomach feel better. I would be lying if I did not admit that I have written up this dietary program, as much because of personal feelings about the ingredients as based upon my conviction in the evidence that has been amassed.

Whether someone follows a particular diet, not only depends on if they *think that it is a good idea* - after being satisfied of its scientific validity - but also because they *feel that it is good for them* , from somewhere deep inside. Knowledge of information is not sufficient to bring about actions. You have to feel a certain way - <u>for</u> or <u>against</u> - the ideas that you have heard about. Once we hear from the manifestos of opposing candidates in a political campaign, we certainly can have opinions of them and arrive at some conclusions, but it is only once we *feel* a certain way about the contender that we are actually motivated to go to the polling station and vote for the person or party we feel is right for the position. To an equal degree, I believe that whether you decide to pursue the diet presented here, depends not only on what you *think* of its contents but on how you *feel* about making it part of your life. In the end, a diet affects how you live every day, so you have to be okay with making a few simple changes – which is easier if you have real belief in what you are doing.

We will always be in search of a cure for one illness or another: a pill that will kill off a bacterial infection, a vaccine that will prevent a pathogen from infecting us in the first place – the purpose of medicine is to find those cures, a task which has been accelerated and improved by the incredible levels of today's technologies. Ultimately, however, my own belief is that Health is the purpose and goal of medical science – in fact, my simple-minded attitude after all is said and done, is that *the Ultimate Cure of Illness is Health*. One doctor – Elinor Levy – makes clear in her popular book on the human being's immune system that: *"no wonder drug can replace the brilliant performance of an effective immune system"*. These are comments which I think would draw the agreement of most immunologists and professors of infectious diseases globally. Maybe one day, food and drink will be considered the central way in which to achieve that – although pills, vaccines, radiation and numerous technologies, are still sure to have an enormous role to play across the spectrum of human treatments. Perhaps all that is needed, is for Science to finally answer the question, conclusively: *how much can diet truly achieve in terms of enabling us to deter Disease and attain Health?*

This is where I must leave things at this stage of **AVD**, for that final question is not mine to answer – only the Future can do that. It is about time to consider the evidence that already exists regarding the anti-viral and immune-system enhancing properties of 52 ingredients at the heart of this diet.

A FOOTNOTE: <u>IN DANGER OF DISMISSAL</u>

ALTHOUGH IT IS MY BELIEF that it is not unwarranted to turn to science for the basis of an anti-viral diet, I am concerned that some people will be put off even considering the idea due to certain articles run by the press. For instance, the Reuters news agency published an article on 27th April 2020 (signed by 'Reuters Staff') called 'False claim: 12 herbs and spices can prevent or treat different viruses'. It is worth taking a look at this for a moment as it does raise some relevant issues.

As far as the context of this online piece is concerned, it is in answer to a post on Facebook entitled 'anti viral herbs' which made the claim that 12 herbs and spices can prevent or treat a variety of illnesses. I have not been able to find the original piece online, so I am assuming it has been removed. Overall, the authors for Reuters rely upon a statement from the website of the National Institutes of Health, which says:

"*The media has reported that some people are seeking "alternative" remedies to prevent infection with the new coronavirus or to treat COVID-19. Some of these purported remedies include herbal therapies and teas. There is no scientific evidence that any of these alternative remedies can prevent or cure COVID-19.*"

I do not know whether the NIH will be updating their remarks any time soon, but research into potential treatments and cures for COVID-19 - including nature-based molecules from herbs and spices - has been moving along at a frantic rate since the start of 2020. As you will see from over 1000 articles relied upon in **Part 2** [*qv.* online database] - one third of references relate to the properties of natural chemicals that can disarm the SARS-CoV-2 virus via a wide variety of bio-molecular mechanisms. - Evidence that *some* natural compounds may be able to prevent or cure COVID-19 *is emerging steadily* - what they need, is to be carefully evaluated.

Sadly, desperation breeds excess and the press as well as social media have been ready to post remarks that are too definitive to be true for long, because scientific research is in such a state of flux. Both results and conclusions from scientific research are liable to misunderstanding and misinterpretation – so that what start out as valid proposals for compounds that *might* defeat COVID-19 *in vivo* as well, become this week's 'New Cure for Covid-19', then being peremptorily debunked by the journalists or news shows as the "next false claim".

From all appearances, the Facebook post discussed by Reuters must have been proposing that people could rely on herbs and spices *alone* and that there is no need for vaccines any more – as they spend most of their piece confirming what are the current, confirmed vaccines for each of the illnesses that natural cures are claimed. And this is all very well as it is foolhardy to suggest that successful medical cures be ignored. Taking one of the natural elements as an example, they rightly quote the CDC's current standard treatment for the diseases for which Garlic has been named as a preventive measure – for example, those immunizations available for HPV (Human Papilloma Virus) and Influenza viruses (offered seasonally).

However, though I believe they are serving a valuable purpose by putting online claims in check – too many of which are unverified, even reckless – Reuters's conclusion that "*These herbs and spices do not prevent or treat infections*" may be a bridge further than scientists would be willing to go concerning the full list of ingredients in question: Oregano, Licorice, Holy Basil, Garlic, Ginger, Fennel, Lemon Balm, Elderberry, Peppermint, Rosemary, Echinacea and Dandelion. All one of those ingredients have been included in the present diet somehow, as my belief is that the balance of scientific evidence has been tipped in their favour. Returning to our example of Garlic, though, I can understand why the CDC have stated that there is "*not enough evidence to show whether garlic is helpful for the common cold*" – as there is only a small amount of research available in that case. However, I think that the NIH is going too far when it writes: *"A great deal of research has been done on garlic, but much of it consists of small, preliminary, or low-quality studies"*. I think that you will find that even the selection of only 20 articles posted in the **AVD** online resource are of more than minor significance.

In the case of Allicin, the active component within garlic, much more research must certainly be done - both in terms of what viruses it neutralizes, what symptoms it can alleviate, even what illnesses it may cure - but enough evidence already supports it being a valid component in therapeutic options. Though I will be first to agree that the evidence varies enormously, in terms of the amount of virus-specific research projects that have been undertaken on the variety of dietary ingredients here - I think that the question is not *if* the natural chemicals in this book have therapeutic effects, but how to ingest them so as to gain the maximum level of viral protection (whether they are fresh or dry, in solid or liquid form *etc.*).

Considering another news channel for a moment, the BBC has been broadcasting a series of 'Coronavirus Health Myths to Ignore' since March 2020, which began with "Myth number one: Eat garlic to avoid infection". The only argument used by them - in this case and with most of the other claims it explores - is to quote the World Health Organization. Chris Morris tells us that *"the WHO says that there is no evidence that eating garlic, or anything else, has protected people from COVID-19"*. However, the main reason why this can be stated so boldly is because no significant amount of clinical trials have yet been undertaken with Garlic, or its bio-active compound Allicin, on SARS-CoV-2. As long as there is an imbalance of research into phytochemicals and pharmaceutical, it is likely that there will also *continue to be* a lack of clinical evidence, although in some areas this has now accumulated to a degree that one can say that the absence of a whole host of dietary micronutrients decreases immunity in general.

Another 'myth' that the BBC were quick to demolish was that: "Lemon Juice protects you from COVID-19". However, once the detailed evidence regarding Vitamin C, Rutin, Naringenin, Hesperidin and Limonene - all of which are present in lemon juice - is properly reviewed, the medical community may wish to give citric fruits some additional attention. The way that media posts can spread like wildfire though, and how uncorroborated half-truths are presented as magic cures just so that a media account can garner looks and likes - *that is in need of being curbed and carefully controlled.* 'Lemon Juice' is not the solution. Discovering a diet that will support an optimum state of health - as a general factor, that- may be of benefit to health services worldwide, because at the present many are being pushed beyond breaking-point.

In such a fast-moving environment, where the results of tests and trials can be announced at a moment's notice, a space of one week can be the difference between the conclusive results from clinical trials being published and an effective vaccine being available. Seeing that pharmaceutical laboratories, as much as academic research facilities, are continuing to undertake intensive investigation into a wide spectrum of nature molecules - some of which have been found to inhibit the SARS-CoV-2 viruses more effectively than any synthetic molecules - the findings of such research will be of just as much relevance to dietary interventions as to pharmaceutical solutions. How bioavailable a compound is when it is ingested as a food, pill or liquid; how quickly it metabolizes in our bodies; what dosage would be necessary in humans - these crucial areas of research can go just as far towards supporting the basis of a diet as to validating a medication.

My discussion has led here because of my concern that media - both online and in print - be more balanced in reporting on matters about the potential of natural ingredients. At the moment, perhaps due to high degrees of anxiety and interest surrounding COVID-19, the press has been in a state of over-excitement. Some damage has been done by shutting down valuable topics which – as far as science is concerned – should be left open. Bizarrely, on the one hand I have witnessed the media in a state of hyperactivity about Vitamin K – based on a single study of its effect on SARS-CoV-2 *in vitro* – while the voluminous quantity of completed research on other naturally occurring chemicals remains almost entirely ignored. Due to its micro-presence in some cheeses, UK paper The Guardian was ready to run with the headline 'Vitamin K found in some cheeses could help fight Covid-19'.

When you add in the overwhelming effect that such news items can have – especially if broadcast with a charismatic presenter and the audience-credibility of a popular show – it is easy to see the dangerous amount of sway that the media can have, whether what they present is true or false.

Too often, the scientists' actual work – experiments they have undertaken, analysis that has taken place, even the conclusions they have reached – is lost amid the noise and we don't find the facts till we search later on. It's easy to get put off Green Tea *today* because a post says it's not healthy – it takes reading research *later* to find out the benefits of EGCG. In my opinion, press writers over the last hundred years have not done enough to reveal to the public the full impact that literally thousands of major results have had on food sciences. Our understanding of Nutrition has made a quantum leap.

As far as the current publication is concerned, I would like to emphasize that the research it is based on – as a whole – extends back to articles that were published half a century ago all the way up to pieces that are being released in journals between September 2020 to January 2021. Remaining as current as possible in terms of its research base is essential to the accuracy of **AVD** – it is being updated continually so as to stay up-to-date with developments and advances in science.

* * * * *

PART 1   A NEW DIET
KEY POINTS

1. *Food Science reveals the connection between good Nutrition and better Immunity, while Chemistry reveals the possibility of Natural Anti-Viral Ingredients*

2. *The Evidence of the connection between Diet and Immunity is ever-increasing - and the idea of an Anti-Viral Diet is rational*

3. *The Emergence of SARS-CoV-2 has now presented us with a serious Viral Threat - especially the disease COVID-19*

4. *There are Lessons to learn from SARS and MERS - especially the use of similar Containment Measures*

5. *Numerous Potential Treatments are being researched, some of which are being helped along by looking at Progress with SARS and MERS*

6. *A Diet that defends against Viruses and Viral Illnesses is a Hypothesis supported by significant Scientific Evidence*

7. *An Anti-Viral Diet is a Viable Option at this moment in time - for Natural Viral Protection*

PART 2

the anti-viral diet

8. THE RIGHT DIET

9. DIETARY HAZARDS

10. THE INGREDIENTS

52 <u>AVD</u> Ingredients

VITAMINS

MINERALS

NUTRIENTS

FLAVONOIDS

HERBS & SPICES

PLANTS & FLOWERS

GASTRO-MODULATORS

OTHER PHYTOCHEMICALS

PART 2

the anti-viral diet

8. THE RIGHT DIET

NOW THAT WE HAVE surveyed the basis of this anti-viral diet in a general manner, it is time to get down to specifics – and this begins by identifying the core of ingredients of the diet. I say 'core', because I do not want you to think that because certain ingredients have not been included in **Part 2** of this book, that they are not important. That is not the case. In a moment, I will try to clarify what has determined whether an ingredient has been included in this part of the book.

As far as this edition of **AVD** is concerned, no argument is being engaged in regarding the general recommended elements of a human diet. The correct balance of dietary ingredients is included at the following informative page on the World Health Organization's website:

www.who.int/news-room/fact-sheets/detail/healthy-diet

The WHO sets out in considerable detail their guidelines for a generally healthy diet – one that will:

"*protect against malnutrition in all its forms, as well as noncommunicable diseases (NCDs), including such as diabetes, heart disease, stroke and cancer.*"

They make the key, essential point that an "*Unhealthy diet and lack of physical activity are leading global risks to health*", then explain in a common-sense manner how different elements of our daily diet should be balanced with each other and how our diet overall should balance with our activities: for example - energy intake with energy expenditure.

When you read this stage of **AVD** therefore, I want you to bear in mind that these general guidelines are the background recommendations of the current diet. They provide a scientifically corroborated basis upon which any healthy diet can rely. Each of the statements about dietary elements made there (about fruit and vegetables, fats, salts, sugars, calories *et alia*) are based upon the findings of food science, nutritional studies and dietetics - above all from the last 50 years.

I would like to emphasize that in terms of highlighting fruit and vegetables as essential ingredients of a healthy diet, WHO are already sending you in the direction of some of the core ingredients of an anti-viral diet. For fruit and vegetables contain many of the vitamins, minerals, other micronutrients and flavonoids - which not only support the immune system but some of which may also have direct anti-viral effects upon viruses. The advice about fruit and vegetables recommends:

> "*always including vegetables in meals;*
> *eating fresh fruit and raw vegetables as snacks;*
> *eating fresh fruit and vegetables that are in season; and*
> *eating a variety of fruit and vegetables.*"

If that is what you do already, then you have already gone some way towards protecting yourself from illnesses, both bacterial and viral. Focusing on variety and freshness of fruit and vegetables is a key directive. Recent research particularly supports the benefits of consuming *raw* vegetables - where edible - and eating fresh fruit. Findings across a range of studies have revealed that we are more likely to receive a larger amount of plants' nutrients when they are raw or fresh, than we would do after cooking or other types of preparation.

Adhere to the general guidelines of WHO's fact sheet on 'Healthy Diet' (whose most recent version is dated 29th April 2020) and your overall diet will be on the right tracks.

However, what we are going to do in this book is to move beyond fundamental advice on what it is healthy to eat - for overall well-being - and focus on what it is advisable to consume in order to deter viruses and their illnesses. In a moment, we are going to survey the range of fifty-two ingredients that have been identified as of importance in this regard. However, I wish to make it clear here that the lack of inclusion of a number of other valuable ingredients does not mean that they are not of significance or have been forgotten. There are a few reasons why a *comprehensive* anti-viral diet - including all potential anti-viral ingredients - is not provided here.

Firstly, unless this book were to become the length of 'War and Peace', it would be impossible to present every individual ingredient about which we have gained knowledge of anti-viral and/or immune-supportive properties. Instead, I have made the choice of including a range of core ingredients which are as representative as possible. Not every beneficial vitamin, mineral and flavonoid, for example, could possibly be included in a book intended for quick, easy reference.

However, in the *second* place, the choice of ingredients in **AVD** have been based upon one requirement more than any other - that a convincing body of evidence exist in support of the qualities that are being indicated for them. In no instance has a dietary element been included where there was not a substantial amount of research behind the purported anti-viral qualities or immuno-modulatory properties.

Thirdly, as this is the first and not the final edition of **AVD** - and is a preliminary attempt at presenting an anti-viral diet which may develop and transform greatly over the years as the results of new research are gathered - it has not been thought necessary to present something comprehensive, final and complete. The idea of an anti-viral diet is something that is in development - not an exhausted area of exploration.

Before we consider 'Version 1.0' of **AVD**, it is important that we mention a few hazards to avoid within this diet.

9. DIETARY HAZARDS

AS THE FOCUS HERE IS ON the elements which you need to *include* in your diet, rather than those that you should *exclude*, we are only going to take a brief moment to look at some of the most important dangers to avoid in order to make sure that you are not taking one step forwards and two steps back – just through not realizing the detrimental effect that certain everyday factors may have upon your general state of health.

The purpose of this diet, as emphasized throughout, is to aim towards better anti-viral protection through the foods that you eat, but also significantly through what you do not eat and by avoiding certain behaviours. In particular, those daily activities that are most likely to decrease your immunity, are obviously ones to be avoided. I am only going to mention five dietary dangers to stay away from – and when I use the word 'dietary' here, it is meant more in terms of an overall way of life and not just relating to what you eat and drink.

Firstly, in terms of what you do consume, it is important to underline the importance of not eating too much of the **wrong fats or oils**. Detailed advice on this is indeed recorded in the WHO guidelines, with their key recommendation being that: "*the intake of saturated fats be reduced to less than 10% of total energy intake and trans-fats to less than 1% of total energy intake*". This is important because it has been shown, in a sizeable amount of research, that obesity – even being over-weight – decreases effectiveness of the immune system. When that happens, you are more prone to viral infections.

Secondly, in a related point, as **excess sugar intake** is also a determining factor in weight gain and obesity, it is vital that you do not exceed the WHO recommendations which are that: "*In both adults and children, the intake of free sugars should be reduced to less than 10% of total energy intake*".

The reason for this is the same as in the previous case – that an excess of fat in the body results in a decrease of immune response. WHO adds that: *"A reduction to less than 5% of total energy intake would provide additional health benefits"*.

In the *third* place, **alcohol** must be mentioned as a factor that can impact the functioning of your immune system. This is not to say that a single drink will suppress your level of immunity. However, research confirms that even three alcohol-containing drinks per day will affect the ability of your white blood cells (which are responsible for fighting off illnesses and infection) to respond in the best way to pathogens. An article such as 'Alcohol, Immunomodulation and Disease' published in Alcohol and Alcoholism (1994) confirmed this early on.

Fourthly, one obvious additional danger to add to this short list is that of **smoking**. Cigarette smoking, as is well established, has harmful effects on the lungs. This includes affecting the macrophages there (a type of white blood cell), which become unable to fight off viruses, bacteria and cancer cells. As in the case of alcohol, this danger has been known of for decades. A valuable article entitled 'Cigarette Smoking influences Cytokine Production and Antioxidant Defences', confirming this danger, was published in Clinical Science (1995).

And *lastly* – though this does not mean there are no more dangers to mention – almost all **recreational drugs** do suppress immunity in one way or another. Cocaine has been shown to cause lack of immune system response and the inability of certain white blood cells to kill pathogens. Heroin, morphine and methadone all cause misfunctioning of the immune system; while marijuana, though less immunosuppressive than all the other mind-altering drugs, does diminish the ability of Natural Killer Cells and decrease Interferon levels.

For more details on all the above dietary dangers and a number of others, visit: www.theantiviraldiet.com/hazards.

10. <u>THE INGREDIENTS</u>

HAVING EXPLAINED the basis for this diet in **Part 1**, there is little need for more of an introduction to the main idea of <u>**AVD**</u>. You are possibly also already aware of the 8 groups of ingredients that we are going to look at, as these are indicated in the Pagefinder. The present (and longest) section of this book, will now proceed to provide essential information about each of the anti-viral ingredients being proposed in this diet. Above all, each individual entry will indicate the way in which that ingredient serves an anti-viral purpose and reference will be made to existing evidence of its properties - a <u>web-link</u> being provided to the supplementary research dossier in each case.

Before each group of dietary ingredients, I have a few words to say about what they have in common and what a few of their key benefits are - in most cases saying little of their anti-viral traits as these are covered in individual entries. We turn first to the best known micronutrients of all - the Vitamins.

VITAMINS

VITAMINS ARE a group of micronutrients that are essential in sufficient quantities for optimal functioning of the body. These chemicals cannot be synthesized within our bodies - at least not in the required amounts - so they must be obtained through our diets. The majority of vitamins are not in fact single molecules, but rather groups of closely related compounds called 'Vitamers'. Altogether there are 13 Vitamins (if Choline is excluded), all of which are essential for the human body to be in a top state of health. These are: Vitamin A (including pro-Vitamin A carotenoids), Vitamin B^1 (thiamine), Vitamin B^2 (riboflavin), Vitamin B^3 (niacin), Vitamin B^5 (pantothenic acid), Vitamin B^6 (pyridoxine), Vitamin B^7 (biotin), Vitamin B^9 (folic acid or folate), Vitamin B^{12} (cobalamins), Vitamin C (ascorbic acid), Vitamin D (calciferols), Vitamin E (tocopherols and tocotrienols) and Vitamin K (phylloquinone and menaquinones).

The vitamins are vital chemicals in many ways, and at least ten Nobel Prizes have been awarded to scientists for discovering them and investigating their special qualities. The *A Vitamins*, for example, regulate the growth of cell and tissue growth; *Vitamin C* and *E* act as antioxidants; *Vitamin D* regulates metabolism of minerals in the bones (and other organs) while the *B Vitamins* are responsible for cell metabolism.

I would like to clarify two words that it is ideal to understand at this point, as they do come up at numerous points in this volume: Firstly, as multiple chemical reactions take place in our bodies, a process called oxidation results in leftover chemicals - like debris, if you will - remaining in our systems. The '*anti-oxidants*' serve the role of scavenging for all those remainder molecules (called 'Free Radicals') and this cleanses our bodies of the harmful remains. As for '*metabolism*', this refers to a group of chemical interactions that are responsible for sustaining our human lives - which includes converting food into intra-cellular energy, turning food into the basis for proteins, lipids, nucleic acids, and carbohydrates - and also processes eliminating the waste chemicals from our bodies.

However, although the vitamins from A to E are known to fulfill a large family of functions, their inclusion in the present diet is based upon their abilities to give extra support to the human immune system and - as a result - exert indirect anti-viral effects upon pathogens. Vitamins B^6, C and E have for some time now been recognized for the contribution they make to the body's system of immunity, with deficiencies in any of them being related to decreased immune response. However, convincing evidence has accumulated regarding the roles that Vitamins A and D - as well as other B Vitamins - play within the body's protective defence mechanisms.

The following five ingredients, therefore, are an essential part of the anti-viral diet. Vitamin K has not been included here, as insufficient scientific evidence exists of its effect upon viruses, though it does appear to suppress some inflammation.

53

Ingredient #1 VITAMIN A

a. Found in:

Beef & Lamb Liver, Liver Sausage, Cod Liver Oil, King Mackerel, Salmon, Bluefin Tuna & Cheddar

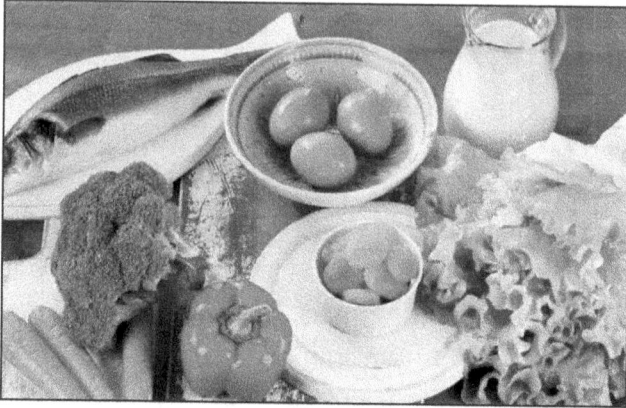

b. Other Sources include:

*Other Cheeses (Limburger, Roquefort, Camembert, Feta **et al.**), Butter, Hard-boiled Egg, Trout & Caviar*

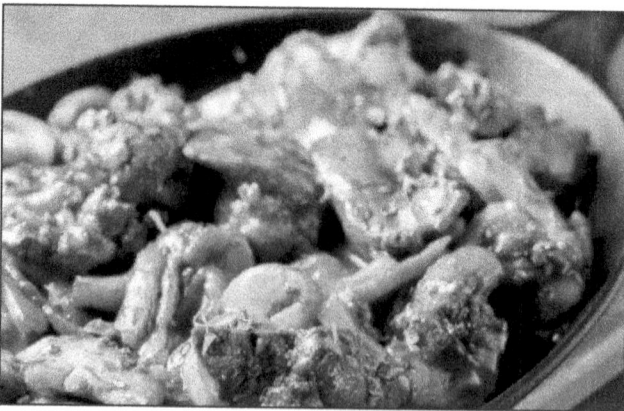

c. Also Found as:

*'Pro-Vitamin A' - Alpha & **Beta-Carotene** [qv. Ingr.#15]*

d. Effect upon Viruses:
Anti-Viral Action evidenced against Norovirus, Influenza, Moloney Sarcoma Virus, Poxvirus & Coxsackievirus A16

e. Impact on Immune System:
Increases Immune Response; Helps Create B- & T-Cells

f. Additional Information:
Powerful Antioxidant; Contributes to Health of Vision. It is currently being researched **re:** SARS-CoV-2 Virus

g. Recommended Daily Intake:
Adults - 800 mcg per day

h. Human Safety:
Non-Toxic within RDI Guidelines / Food is Safest Source

i. Research Quote - Immuno-Enhancing Effects:
"Vitamin A supplementation to infants has shown the potential to improve antibody response after some vaccines, including measles and anti-rabies vaccination (2.1 times). In addition an enhanced immune response to influenza virus vaccination has also been observed in children (2–8 years) who were vitamin A and D-insufficient at baseline, after supplementation with vitamin A and D." [1]

j. Research Quote - Potential Effect on COVID-19:
"The mechanism by which vitamin A and retinoids inhibit measles replication is upregulating elements of the innate immune response in uninfected bystander cells, making them refractory to productive infection during subsequent rounds of viral replication. Therefore, vitamin A could be a promising option for the treatment of this novel coronavirus and the prevention of lung infection." [2]

k. Online Dossier of Scientific Research Findings:
https://theantiviraldiet.com/ingredient-%231-%2B-research

Ingredient #2 VITAMIN B

a. Found in:

Salmon, Leafy Greens, Liver and Other Organ Meats, Eggs, Milk, Beef, Oysters, Clams, Mussels & Legumes

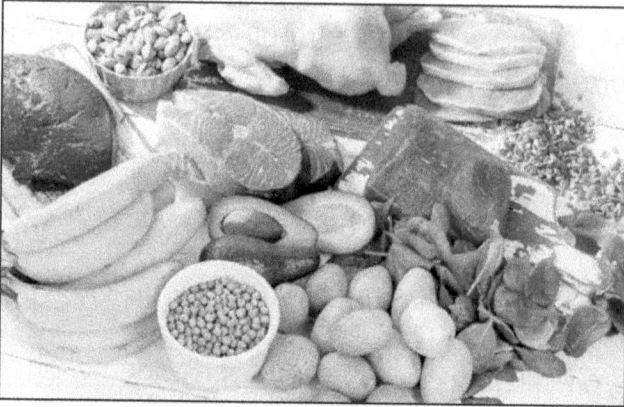

b. Other Sources include:

Chicken, Turkey, Yogurt, Nutritional/Brewer's Yeast Pork, Fortified Cereals, Trout & Sunflower Seeds

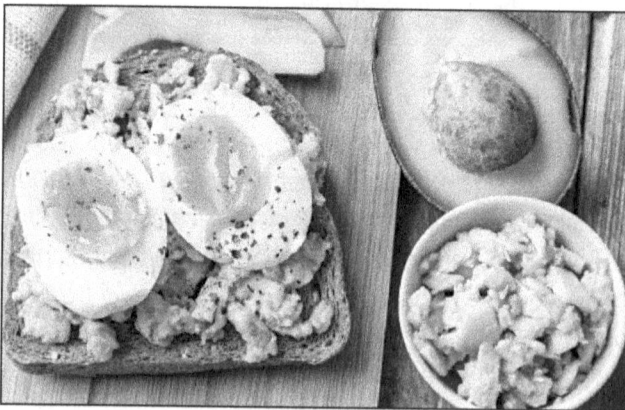

c. Consists of:

A Group of 8 Vitamers: B^1, B^2, B^3, B^5, B^6, B^7, B^9 & B^{12}

d. Effect upon Viruses:
Anti-Viral Action evidenced against Hepatitis C *inter alia*

e. Impact on Immunity:
Increases Immune Response; B^6 helps produce Cytokines and Lymphocytes (which increase Immune Response)

f. Additional Information:
B^6 is also an Antioxidant; Lack of B^9 & B^{12} causes Anemia

g. Recommended Daily Intake:
Adults: B^1 - 1.4 mg; B^2 - 1.6 mg; B^3 - 18 mg; B^5 - 6 mg; B^6 - 2 mg; B^7 - 30 mcg; B^9 - 400 mcg; B^{12} - 6 mcg.

h. Human Safety:
Non-Toxic within RDI Guidelines / Food is Safest Source

i. Research Quote – Immuno-Supportive Effect:
"[...] *an array of micronutrients are required to meet the complex needs of the immune system, including vitamins A, D, C, E,* **B6, B12**, *folate, copper, iron, zinc and selenium, with many of these having potential synergistic relationships.*" [3]

j. Research Quote – Potential Effect on COVID-19:
"*Moreover, vitamin B3 treatment significantly inhibited neutrophil infiltration into the lungs with a strong anti-inflammatory effect during ventilator-induced lung injury. However, it also paradoxically led to the development of significant hypoxemia. Vitamin B6 is also needed in protein metabolism and it participates in over 100 reactions in body tissues. In addition, it also plays important role in body immune function as well. As shortage of B vitamins may weaken host immune response, they should be supplemented to the virus-infected patients to enhance their immune system. Therefore, B vitamins could be chosen as a basic option for the treatment of COVID-19.*" [2]

k. Online Dossier of Scientific Research Findings:
https://theantiviraldiet.com/ingredient-%232-%2B-research

Ingredient #3 VITAMIN C

a. Found in:

Kakadu Plum, Acerola Cherry, Rose Hip, Chili Peppers, Guava, Sweet Yellow Peppers, Blackcurrants & Thyme

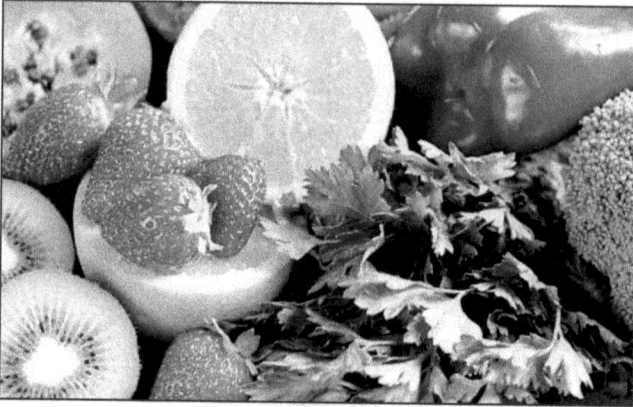

b. Other Sources include:

Parsley, Mustard Spinach, Kale, Kiwi, Broccoli, Brussels Sprouts, Lychees, Persimmons, Strawberries & Papaya

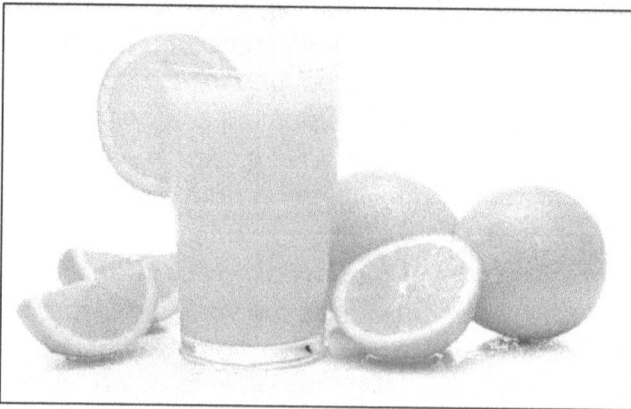

c. Most Common Source:

As Orange Juice (ideally Pressed) - Popular Worldwide

d. Effect upon Viruses:
Anti-Viral Action evidenced against Norovirus & Influenza

e. Impact on Immunity:
Increases Immune Response by contributing to Cellular Functions of the Innate and Adaptive Immune Systems

f. Additional Information:
Vitamin C is also known as 'Ascorbic Acid' or 'Ascorbate'. It is currently being researched **re:** SARS-CoV-2 Virus

g. Recommended Daily Intake:
Adults - 80 mg per day (Women: 75 mg / Men: 90 mg)

h. Human Safety:
Non-Toxic within RDI Guidelines / Food is Safest Source

i. Research Quote - Anti-Viral & Immune Effects:
"There is evidence that vitamin C and quercetin co-administration exerts a synergistic antiviral action due to overlapping antiviral and immunomodulatory properties and the capacity of ascorbate to recycle quercetin, increasing its efficacy. Safe, cheap interventions which have a sound biological rationale should be prioritized for experimental use in the current context of a global health pandemic." [4]

j. Research Quote - Potential Effect on COVID-19:
"Three human controlled trials had reported that there was significantly lower incidence of pneumonia in vitamin C- supplemented groups, suggesting that vitamin C might prevent the susceptibility to lower respiratory tract infections under certain conditions. The COVID-19 had been reported to cause lower respiratory tract infection, so vitamin C could be one of the effective choices for the treatment of COVID-19." [2]

k. Online Dossier of Scientific Research Findings:
https://theantiviraldiet.com/ingredient-%233-%2B-research

Ingredient #4 VITAMIN D

a. <u>Found in</u>:

Salmon, Herring, Sardines, Mackerel, Cod Liver Oil, Canned Tuna, Beef Liver, Egg Yolks & Mushrooms

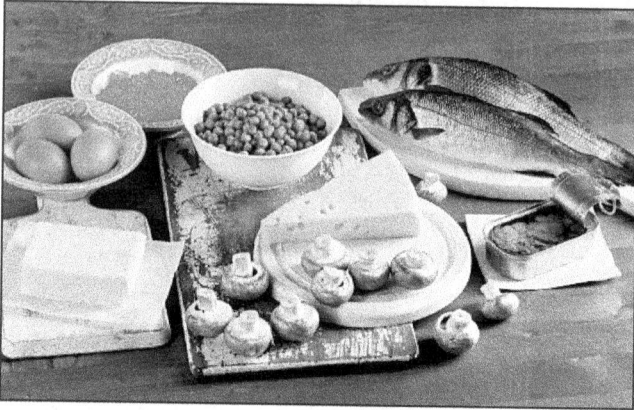

b. <u>Other Sources include</u>:

Cheese (Fontina, Muenster, Monterey) and Fortified Foods: Cow's Milk, Soy Milk, Orange Juice & Cereals

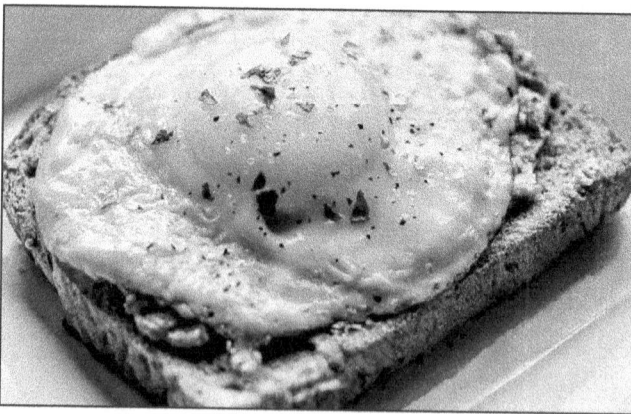

c. <u>Essential for</u>:

*The Absorption of Vitamin D - **viz.** for Bone Strength*

d. Effect upon Viruses:
Indirectly, by Stimulation of the Immune System *qv.* **e.**

e. Impact on Immunity:
Improves the Innate and Adaptive Immune Responses.
Deficiency results in Greater Susceptibility to Infection

f. Additional Information:
In Vitro experiments (*eg* with Bronchial Epithelial Cells)
show that Vitamin D may have Direct Anti-Viral Effects

g. Recommended Daily Intake:
Adults – 5 mcg per day

h. Human Safety:
Non-Toxic within RDI Guidelines / Food is Safest Source

i. Research Quote – Effects on SARS-CoV-2:
"*In summary, we postulate that conventional oral vitamin D supplementation can be a ready strategy to aim: (i) restriction of SARS-CoV-2 infection via downregulation of ACE2 receptor, and (ii) attenuation of disease severity by down-tuning the pulmonary pro-inflammatory response or cytokine storm that fuels COVID-19 severity.*" [5]

j. Research Quote – Potential Effect on COVID-19:
"*Daneshkhah and coworkers demonstrated that the age-specific case fatality rate of COVID-19 was highest in Italy, Spain, and France, European countries with the highest incidence severe vitamin D deficiency. Our findings suggest that vitamin D deficiency may partly explain the geographic variations in the reported case fatality rate of COVID-19, implying that supplementation with vitamin D may reduce the mortality from this pandemic.*" [6]

k. Online Dossier of Scientific Research Findings:
https://theantiviraldiet.com/ingredient-%234-%2B-research

Ingredient #5 VITAMIN E

a. Found in:

Wheatgerm Oil, Sunflower Seeds, Almonds, Almond Oil
Mamey Sapote, Sunflower Oil, Hazelnut Oil & Hazelnuts

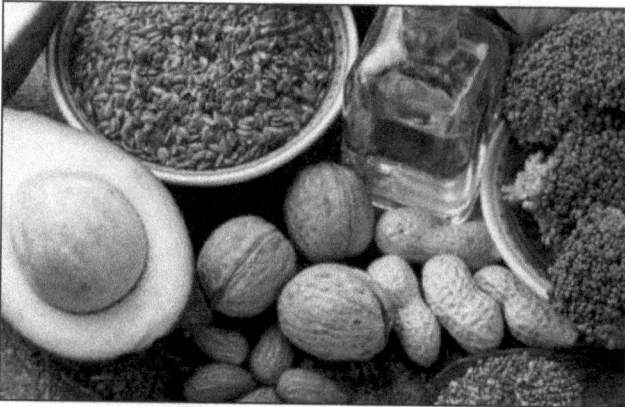

b. Other Sources include:

Abalone, Pine Nuts, Goose Meat, Peanuts, Avocado,
Atlantic Salmon, Rainbow Trout & Red Sweet Peppers

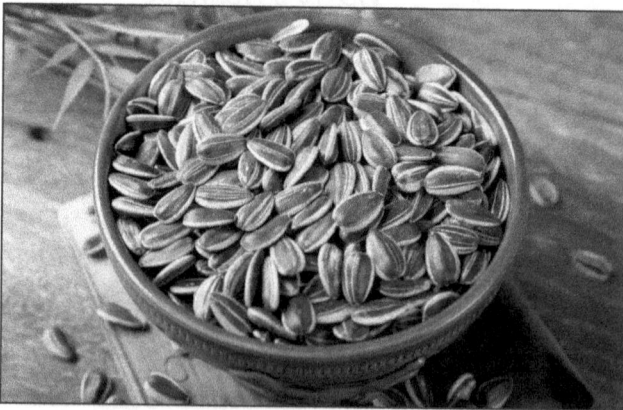

c. Present in:

Most Foods, to a large extent - Vit. E Deficiency is Rare

d. Effect upon Viruses:
Indirectly, by Stimulation of the Immune System *qv.* **e.**

e. Impact on Immunity:
Vital for Optimum Maintenance of the Immune System and crucially Protects against its Age-Related Decline

f. Additional Information:
High Vitamin E Diet addresses the Decreased Levels of Vitamin E in Older People and those having AIDS

g. Recommended Daily Intake:
Adults - 10 mg per day

h. Human Safety:
Non-Toxic within RDI Guidelines / Food is Safest Source

i. Research Quote - Effects upon ARDS:
"*In 3 studies, the authors reported a potential benefit of the intervention on outcomes: intramuscular cholecalciferol on mortality, intramuscular vitamin E on Acute Physiology and Chronic Health Evaluation score in patients with ARDS and zinc sulfate on the incidence of ventilator-associated pneumonia in ventilated patients in intensive care units.*" [6]

j. Research Quote - Effect on Hepatitis B Virus:
"*However positive effects of vitamin E have been observed in the treatment of chronic hepatitis B in a small pilot RCT, where a significantly higher normalization of liver enzymes and HBV-DNA negativization, was observed in the vitamin E group. Similar results have been observed in a RCT in the paediatric population, where vitamin E treatment resulted in a higher anti-HBe seroconversion and virological response.*" [1]

k. Online Dossier of Scientific Research Findings:
https://theantiviraldiet.com/ingredient-%235-%2B-research

MINERALS

IN TERMS OF THE HUMAN BODY, Minerals are those chemical elements that serve as essential nutrients for life functions. Elements are the most basic constituents of all chemical compounds and 118 elements have been identified as of 2020. 96% of the weight of our bodies is accounted for by four elements alone - Oxygen, Hydrogen, Carbon and Nitrogen - and these are not usually included in the list of dietary minerals. The five main minerals in the human body are Calcium, Phosphorus, Potassium, Sodium and Magnesium; however, there are also ten additional minerals that serve important roles in the human system, even though in extremely small amounts. These minerals are known as 'Trace Elements' and should not be ignored just because they are only needed in minuscule quantities. They all serve crucial biochemical functions and are usually listed as: Sulphur, Iron, Chlorine, Cobalt, Copper, Zinc, Manganese, Molybdenum, Iodine and Selenium.

In terms of the minerals that are included in this diet, one of them belongs to the group of five main minerals (Magnesium), five of them are from the group of trace elements above (Zinc, Iron, Manganese, Copper and Selenium), while one of them (Boron) has only recently been appreciated in terms of its importance to human life. The individual entries on these seven minerals focus on their qualities in terms of antiviral effect and immune system support, but here follow a few introductory words on the nature and purpose of each one.

Magnesium, the eleventh most abundant of elements in the human body, is vital to all cells, as well as to around 300 enzymes. These enzymes (which are proteins that help to accelerate biochemical reactions) rely on Magnesium ions in order to function. Magnesium is thus a vital mineral to us.

Zinc is essential to human development - especially important at the pre-natal and post-natal phase. Deficiency in

Zinc at the early stages in life slows down growth and makes one susceptible to illness and disease. Sadly, Zinc deficiency affects almost two billion people in developing countries.

Iron is a vital element to two key processes in the human body: oxygen transport by our blood, plus oxygen storage within our muscles. Only about 4 grams of iron exist in an average adult, mainly in the form of the two proteins hemoglobin and myoglobin. Iron deficiency can have a very detrimental effect on the body – even death – and it also causes anemia.

Manganese - although its exact contributions to bodily functions have only been discovered relatively recently – is essential to support a wide variety of enzymes. It is especially important as an antioxidant in the detoxification of reactive oxygen species in the body, helping to prevent cell damage.

Copper is mainly found in the bones, muscles and livers of humans. It is essential as a key component of the vital respiratory enzyme called 'Cytochrome C Oxidase'. Copper deficiency can be an issue, causing muscle weakness, anemia, connective tissue problems and a low white blood cell count.

Selenium, though only required in micro-quantity, supports several cellular functions - not only in humans but other animals also. Like Manganese, it is a constituent of antioxidant enzymes, which protect the body from cellular damage. Deficiency in Selenium causes numerous health issues, including fatigue, infertility, hair loss and a weakened immunity.

Lastly – *Boron* – though it has not been included in lists of essential minerals, has a wide range of functions. Mentioning only four of these: Boron promotes the growth and maintenance of bone; it improves the healing of wounds; it benefits the body's use of estrogen, testosterone and of vitamin D; and it boosts the body's absorption of Magnesium. Its impact upon the immune system has only recently been discovered.

Although there are other minerals which do have an impact on the body's immune system, it appears from the evidence that these seven elements are the most significant. They have direct effect on immunity and indirectly on anti-virality.

Ingredient #6 ZINC

a. <u>Found in</u>:

Meat (particularly Red Meat), Shellfish, Legumes, Seeds, Nuts, Dairy Products, Eggs & Whole Grains

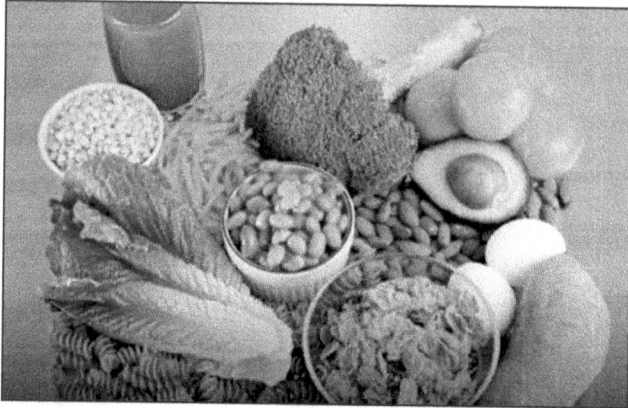

b. <u>Other Sources include</u>:

Dark Chocolate, Firm Tofu, Lentils, Oatmeal, Shiitake Mushrooms, Potatoes, Green Beans, Kale (Low Amounts)

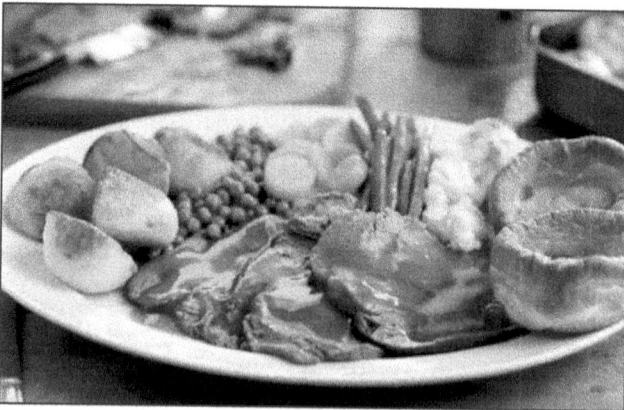

c. <u>Hardly Present in</u>:

Fruit and Vegetables - generally Low Sources of Zinc

d. Effect upon Viruses:
Direct Anti-Viral Action possibly evidenced against Hepatitis E Virus, Respiratory Syncytial Virus & H1N1

e. Impact on Immunity:
Zinc is Essential to the Thymus Gland, where T-Lymphocytes - including the crucial CD4 Cells - are Produced

f. Additional Information:
Zinc Deficiency results in a Weakened Immune Response

g. Recommended Daily Intake:
Adults - 15 mg per day

h. Human Safety:
Non-Toxic within RDI Guidelines / Food is Safest Source

i. Research Quote - Anti-Viral/Viral Replication:
"*Effectiveness of Zn against a number of viral species is mainly realized through the physical processes, such as virus attachment, infection, and uncoating. Zn may also protect or stabilize the cell membrane which could contribute to blocking of the virus entry into the cell. On the other hand, it was demonstrated that Zn may inhibit viral replication.*" [7]

j. Research Quote - Potential against COVID-19:
"*As zinc is essential to preserve natural tissue barriers such as the respiratory epithelium, preventing pathogen entry, for a balanced function of the immune system and the redox system, zinc deficiency can probably be added to the factors predisposing individuals to infection and detrimental progression of COVID-19. Finally, due to its direct antiviral properties, it can be assumed that zinc administration is beneficial for most of the population, especially those with suboptimal zinc status.*" [8]

k. Online Dossier of Scientific Research Findings:
https://theantiviraldiet.com/ingredient-%236-%2B-research

Ingredient #7 IRON

a. <u>Found in</u>:

Beef Liver, Chicken Liver, Clams, Mussels, Oysters, Beef, Chicken, Turkey, Ham, Canned Tuna & Veal

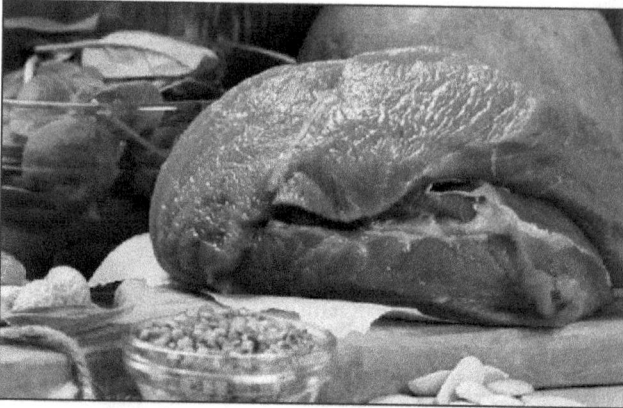

b. <u>Vegetarian Sources include</u>:

Beans, Peas, Lentils, Tofu, Tempeh, Natto, Soybeans, Seeds, Nuts, Leafy Greens, Olives, Quinoa & Spelt

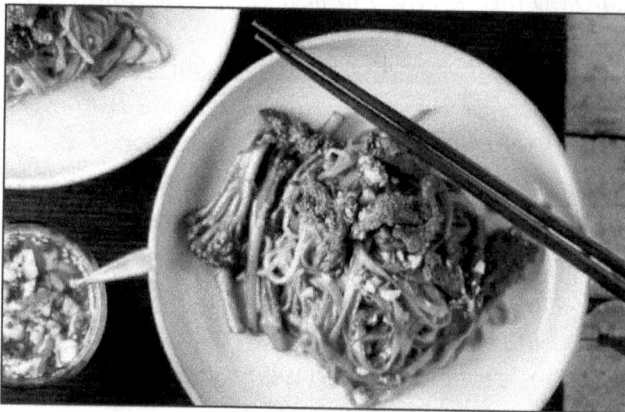

c. <u>Found as</u>:

Heme Iron (Animal Products) & Non-Heme Iron (Plants)

d. Effect upon Viruses:
Indirectly, by Proper Support of the Immune System *qv.* **e.**

e. Impact on Immunity:
Iron is Vital to create a Protein in Red Blood Cells that takes Oxygen from the Lungs to All Parts of the Body. It is also Essential for Innate and Adaptive Immunity. Deficiency can be a Problem, but so can Overload.

f. Additional Information:
Healthy Intake, within Guidelines, needs to be Observed

g. Recommended Daily Intake:
Adults – 15 mg per day

h. Human Safety:
Non-Toxic within RDI Guidelines / Food is Safest Source

i. Research Quote – Iron Levels in COVID-19 Patients:
"Decreased serum iron level could predict the transition of COVID-19 from mild to severe and critical illness. Seven (53.8%) patients with a lower serum iron level after treatment in the critical group had died. There was a significant difference in posttreatment serum iron levels between COVID-19 survivors and non-survivors." [9]

j. Research Quote – Iron Chelation in SARS-CoV-2:
"Emerging studies indicate that iron manipulation, such as iron chelation, is a promising adjuvant therapy in treating viral infection. While the emerging viral infection by SARS-CoV-2 is much less understood compared with HIV-1 or SARS-CoV and MERS-CoV, based on the previous studies, it is plausible that deprivation of iron supply to the virus could serve as a beneficial adjuvant in treating the SARS-CoV-2 infection." [10]

k. Online Dossier of Scientific Research Findings:
https://theantiviraldiet.com/ingredient-%237-%2B-research

Ingredient #8 MAGNESIUM

a. Found in:

Dark Chocolate, Avocado, Almonds, Brazil Nuts,
Cashews, Lentils, Beans, Chickpeas, Soybeans & Tofu

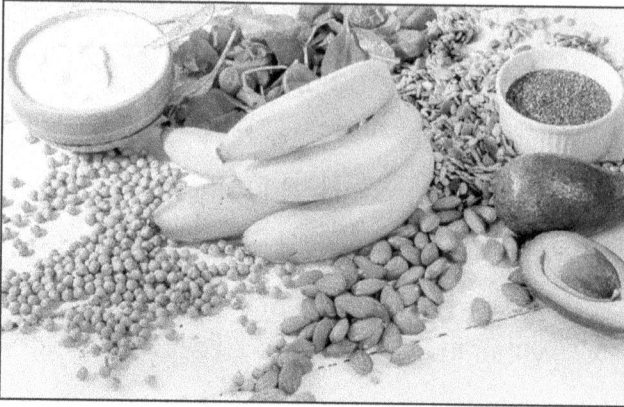

b. Other Sources include:

Flax Seeds, Pumpkin Seeds, Chia Seeds, Wheat, Oats,
Barley, Salmon, Mackerel, Bananas & Leafy Greens

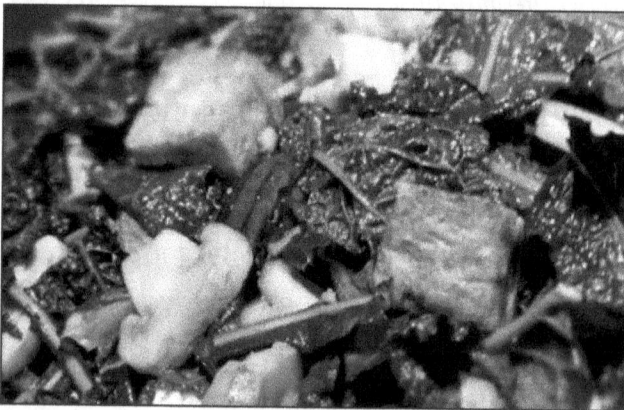

c. It is Noted that:

Foods with Protein may enhance Magnesium Absorption

d. Effect upon Viruses:
Indirectly, through Support of the Immune System *qv.* **e.** though some Research points to direct Anti-Viral Effects

e. Impact on Immunity:
Magnesium is one of 7 Major Minerals in the Human Body – Essential for Strengthening the Immune System

f. Additional Information:
Deficiency can cause Fatigue, Nausea and Vomiting

g. Recommended Daily Intake:
Adults – 350 mg per day

h. Human Safety:
Non-Toxic within RDI Guidelines / Food is Safest Source

i. Research Quote – Significance for COVID-19:
"Clinical recommendations are given for prevention and treatment of COVID-19. Constant monitoring of ionized magnesium status with subsequent repletion, when appropriate, may be an effective strategy to influence disease contraction and progression. The peer-reviewed literature supports that several aspects of magnesium nutrition warrant clinical consideration." [11]

j. Research Quote – Potential against SARS-CoV-2:
"Magnesium (Mg) has a strong relation with the immune system and immunological functions are disturbed in case of Mg deficiency. [...] [I]ntracellular free Mg concentration contributes significantly to antiviral immunity. Therefore, decreased resistance against infection with SARS-CoV-2 in case of Mg deficiency can be assumed. However, there are some more potential connections between Mg and COVID-19 worth mentioning." [12]

k. Online Dossier of Scientific Research Findings:
https://theantiviraldiet.com/ingredient-%238-%2B-research

Ingredient #9 MANGANESE

a. Found in:

Mussels, Toasted Wheat Germ, Firm Tofu, Sweet Potatoes, Pine Nuts, Brown Rice & Lima Beans

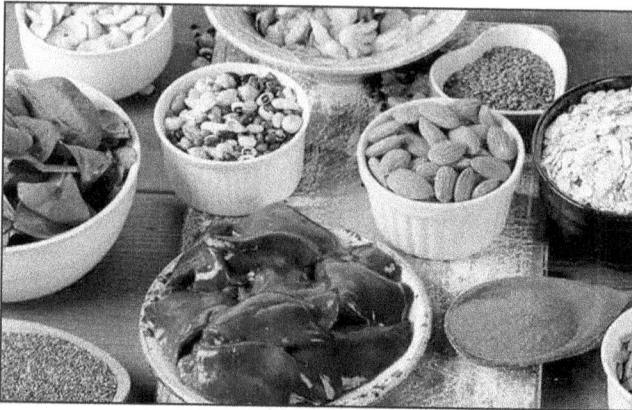

b. Other Sources include:

Chick Peas, Spinach, Pineapple, Lamb Liver, Chicken Liver, Celery Seeds, Poppy Seeds, Cocoa & Hazelnuts

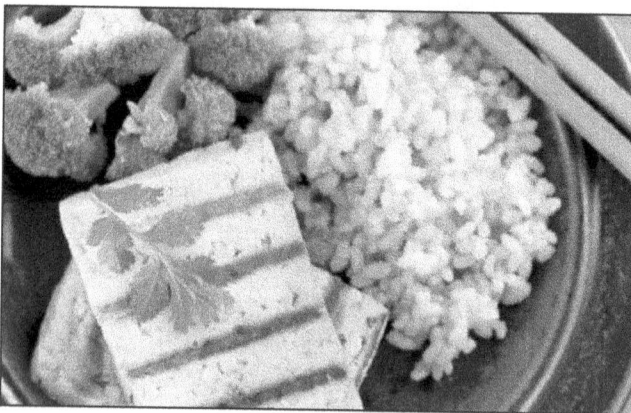

c. You Must Avoid:

Manganese Excess. Toxicity causes Neurological Issues

d. Effect upon Viruses:
Indirectly, by Proper Support of the Immune System *qv.* **e.**

e. Impact on Immunity:
Manganese appears to be of Essential Importance for Intracellular Communication within the Immune System

f. Additional Information:
It is Needed for Healthy Brain Functioning, but only RDI

g. Recommended Daily Intake:
Adults - 5 mg per day

h. Human Safety:
Non-Toxic within RDI Guidelines / Food is Safest Source

i. Research Quote - Anti-Viral Defence Mechanism:
"*Although several parts of the puzzle are still missing, it appears that manganese, or more precisely changes in its cytoplasmic concentration, is one language used by innate immune cells for their intracellular communication. So far, a strong increase of cytosolic Mn2+ in response to viral infection is reported, but it remains unclear what triggers the cell to release Mn2+ from its stores. It would be extremely interesting o identify the receptors, transporters, and other regulatory mechanisms involved in Mn2+ translocation, and evaluate their potential for modifying the body's antiviral defense for therapeutic purposes.*" [13]

j. Research Quote - Importance to Avoid Excess:
"*Unlike zinc, there is little information regarding the effects of manganese deficiency on immune development and function. There are, however, limited data suggesting that toxic levels of manganese may impair immune function.*" [14]

k. Online Dossier of Scientific Research Findings:
https://theantiviraldiet.com/ingredient-%239-%2B-research

Ingredient #10 SELENIUM

a. Found in:

Brazil Nuts, Yellowfin Tuna, Sardines, Oysters, Clams, Halibut, Shrimp, Salmon, Crab, Ham, Pork & Beef

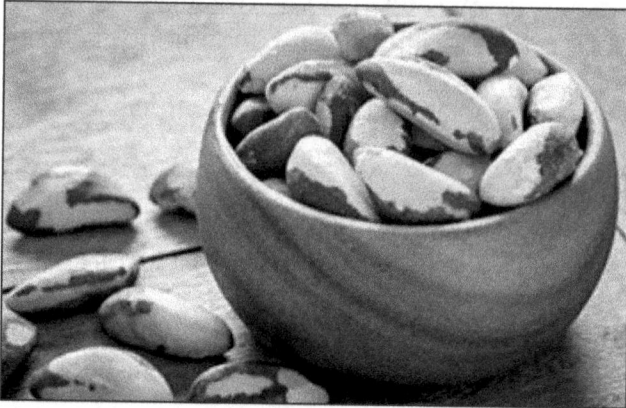

b. Other Sources include:

Turkey, Chicken, Cottage Cheese, Eggs, Brown Rice, Sunflower Seeds, Baked Beans, Mushrooms & Oatmeal

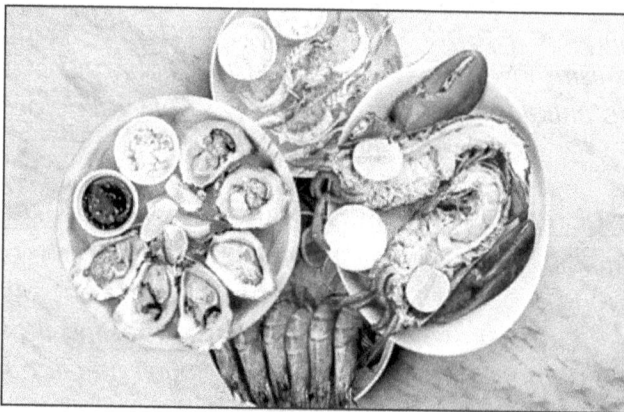

c. Deficiency may cause:

Infertility, Muscle Weakness, Hair Loss and Fatigue

d. Effect upon Viruses:
Indirectly, by Proper Support of the Immune System qv. **e.**

e. Impact on Immunity:
The Health of the Human Immune System significantly relies on Selenium Intake. Without ample, it is weakened

f. Additional Information:
Selenium may be a Key Element in blocking Viral Attack

g. Recommended Daily Intake:
Adults – 35 mcg per day

h. Human Safety:
Non-Toxic within RDI Guidelines / Food is Safest Source

i. Research Quote - COVID-19 Cure Correlation:
"Our results show an association between the reported cure rates for COVID-19 and selenium status. These data are consistent with the evidence of the antiviral effects of selenium from previous studies. Indeed, multiple cellular and viral mechanisms involving selenium and selenoproteins could influence viral pathogenicity." [15]

j. Research Quote - Protection against SARS-CoV-2:
"Therefore, we conclude that Se status is likely to influence human response to the SARS-CoV-2 infection and that Se status is one (of several) risk factors which may impact on the outcome of SARS-CoV-2 infection, particularly in populations where Se intake is sub-optimal or low. We suggest the use of appropriate markers to assess the Se status of COVID-19 patients and possible supplementation may be beneficial in limiting the severity of symptoms, especially in countries where Se status is regarded as sub-optimal." [16]

k. Online Dossier of Scientific Research Findings:
https://theantiviraldiet.com/ingredient-%2310-%2B-research

Ingredient #11 BORON

a. Found in:

Raisins, Almonds, Hazelnuts, Dried Apricots, Brazil Nuts, Peanut Butter, Walnuts, Kidney Beans & Prunes

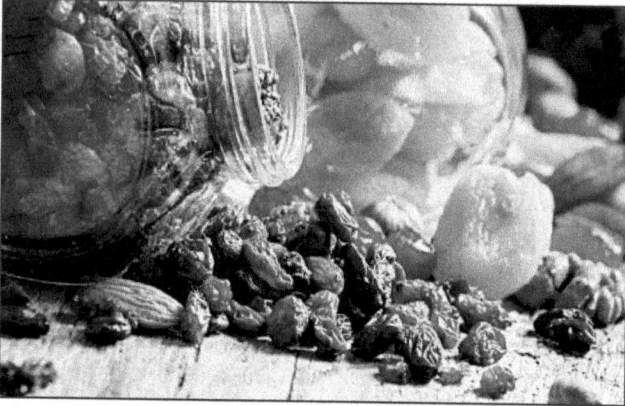

b. Other Sources include:

Raw Cashew Nuts, Dates, Wine (Shiraz Cabernet), Lentils, Chickpeas, Peach, Olives & Bananas

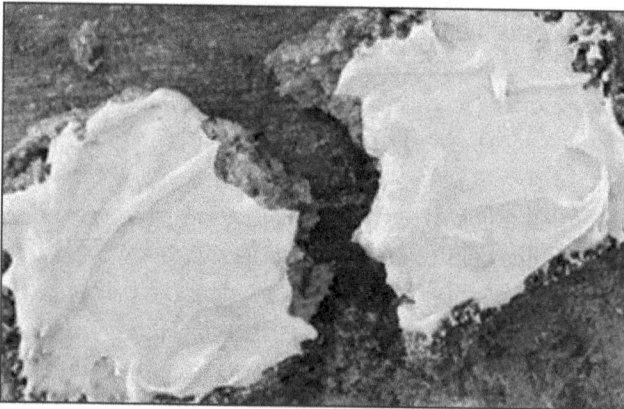

c. Appears to Affect:

How Body handles Calcium, Magnesium & Phosphorus

d. Effect upon Viruses:
Indirectly, by Proper Support of the Immune System *qv.* **e.**

e. Impact on Immunity:
Boron increases the Proliferation of Lymphocytes – one group of White Blood Cells within the Immune System

f. Additional Information:
Boron is a Regulator of Immune & Inflammatory Responses

g. Recommended Daily Intake:
Adults – < 20 mg per day

h. Human Safety:
Non-Toxic within RDI Guidelines / Food is Safest Source

i. Research Quote – The Essentiality of Boron:
"Current research implicates boron as an essential nutrient in humans demonstrating healthful effects in cellular functions associated with osteoporosis, arthritis, inflammation and cancer." [17]

j. Research Quote – Positive Impact of Boron:
"Findings have shown that boron is needed to complete the life cycle of some higher animals; in nutritional amounts, it promotes bone health, brain function, and the immune or inflammatory response; alleviates or decreases the risk for arthritis; facilitates the action or utilization of several hormones; and is associated with decreased risk for some cancers. This suggests that boron intakes above 1 mg/d could help people "live longer and better". Increased intakes of boron through consuming foods such as fruits, vegetables nuts, and pulses should be recognized as a reasonable dietary recommendation." [18]

k. Online Dossier of Scientific Research Findings:
https://theantiviraldiet.com/ingredient-%2311-%2B-research

Ingredient #12 COPPER

a. Found in:

Oysters, Beef Liver, Shiitake Mushrooms, Firm Tofu, Sweet Potato, Sesame Seeds & Dry Roasted Cashews

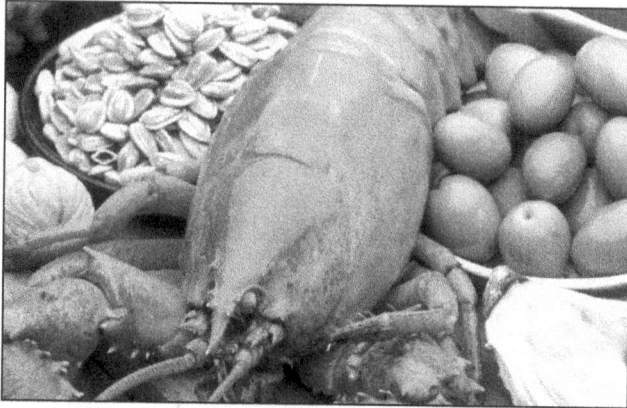

b. Other Sources include:

Chickpeas, Salmon, Lobster, Swiss Chard, Kale, Dark Chocolate, Spinach, Avocado & Sundried Tomatoes

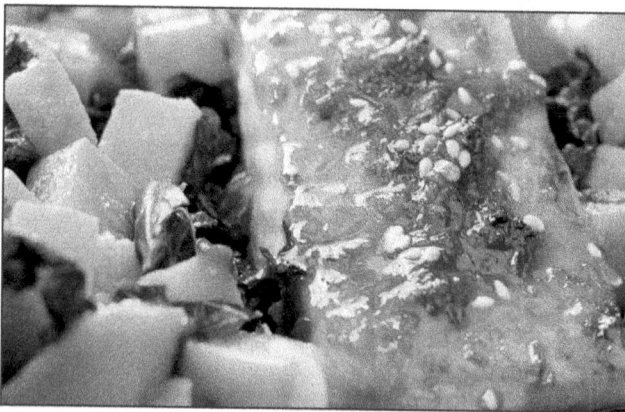

c. Deficiency may cause:

*Muscle Weakness, Anemia & Low WBC Count **et al.***

d. Effect upon Viruses:
Indirectly, by Proper Support of the Immune System qv. **e.**

e. Impact on Immunity:
Copper is Essential for Optimal Functioning of the Innate Immune System. Deficiency causes Weakened Immunity

f. Additional Information:
Copper Kills Numerous Bacteria Directly within the Body

g. Recommended Daily Intake:
Adults – 2 mg per day

h. Human Safety:
Non-Toxic within RDI Guidelines / Food is Safest Source

i. Research Quote – Deficiency and Infectability:
"*However, the most susceptible population to copper deficiency are infants. Gibson (1985) has reported that the intake of copper by breast-fed or formula-fed infants is below the US RDA. Furthermore, tht intake of copper following weaning may be hampered by poor absorption from cells (Bell et al., 1987) and by negative interactions with supplements such as iron (Haschke et al., 1986). During infancy, copper deficiency is often associated with infection as documented in seven separate reports.*" [19]

j. Research Quote – Anti-Viral against Influenza:
"*Copper plays a crucial role in immunity by participating in the development and differentiation of immune cells. In-vitro studies have shown that copper demonstrates antiviral properties. For example, thujaplicin-copper chelates inhibit replication of human influenza viruses, while intracellular copper has been shown to regulate the influenza virus life cycle.*" [1]

k. Online Dossier of Scientific Research Findings:
https://theantiviraldiet.com/ingredient-%2312-%2B-research

NUTRIENTS

THOUGH THIS SUB-SECTION has been entitled 'Nutrients', it is not about nutrients in general but is merely a selection of a handful of special ingredients that have nutritional value, at the same time as being of special use in terms of fighting off viruses and empowering the immune system. The seven main classes of nutrients are of course: Carbohydrates, Fats, Fibre, Minerals, Proteins, Vitamins and Water. Out of these, we have already looked at ingredients taken from two groups of 'micronutrients' – so named because we only need to ingest them in extremely small quantities for them to be beneficial. Other nutrients, which are required in larger quantities – such as the carbohydrates and proteins – are named 'macronutrients'. Those included within this section are a mixture of micro- and macro- nutrients because of the quantities recommended to be consumed as part of a diet. Before surveying their anti-viral /immuno-modulatory qualities, I think that a general knowledge of some of these ingredients' properties will be helpful.

Omega-3 fatty acids or oils, often simply referred to as Omega-3, are polyunsaturated fatty acids (PUFA) – thus of the type approved by WHO – and they play significant roles in the human body. They need to be obtained through diet as they cannot otherwise be synthesized within the body. In terms of benefits, Omega-3 has been shown to lower blood pressure, slow down the development of plaque in the arteries and reduce the likelihood of heart disease and strokes.

Alpha-Lipoic Acid, also known as a-lipoic acid and thioctic acid, is a chemical produced in animals normally, and it is essential for 'aerobic metabolism' – which is the way our bodies create energy through the combustion of carbohydrates, amino acids, and fats in the presence of oxygen. Although it *can* be created in the body and gained from diet, Alpha-Lipoic Acid is also sold as an antioxidant supplement.

The third ingredient in this sub-section, *Beta-Carotene*, is also known as the main dietary source of 'Pro-Vitamin A'. A Pro-Vitamin (or provitamin) is a substance which, within the body, can be converted into a vitamin. β-carotene is the best-known plant carotenoid, found in high quantity in carrots and sweet potato. Good intake of Beta-Carotene is beneficial to skin health, the mucus membranes, vision and immunity.

Beta Glucans - which are a source of soluble, fermentable fibre - have been discovered to have a positive impact on the human body. β-Glucans (beta-glucans) occur naturally in the cell walls of cereals, bacteria and fungi. The type of prebiotic fibre that they provide improves digestive function, blood cholesterol levels and glucose metabolism. Beta-Glucans can reduce the risk of cardiovascular diseases.

L-Carnitine - though perhaps a less well-known nutrient - can be of great health benefit. It occurs naturally in humans and is derived from amino acids. Its name derives from the Latin word for meat (*'carnis'*) as it is found most plentifully in that source. Clinical research indicates that L-Carnitine - like the Beta-Glucans - can alleviate cardiovascular disease. It is not yet proven whether it improves athletic performance and recovery, though research in that area is currently on-going.

It is important to emphasize that this is not a comprehensive list of Nutrients and that these ingredients have only been brought together under this heading as they do not belong in the foregoing categories of Vitamins or Minerals. The nutrients included in this section are those only, for which I have found sufficient proof regarding their anti-viral effects and/or immuno-modulatory properties. There are other candidates to consider - such as N-Acetyl-L-Cysteine and Lycopene - but until the burden of evidence is sufficient they will not be included in this anti-viral diet. For more detailed information on all of the nutrients within this diet - as I have only been providing snapshots here - I would recommend referring to the Encyclopaedia Britannica (www.britannica.com).

Ingredient #13 OMEGA-3

a. <u>Found in</u>:

Mackerel, Salmon, Cod Liver Oil, Herring, Oysters, Sardines, Anchovies, Caviar, Flax Seeds & Chia Seeds

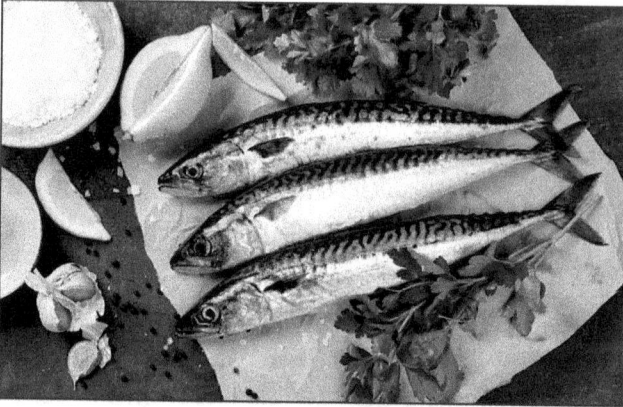

b. <u>Other Sources include</u>:

Walnuts, Soybeans, Hemp Seeds, Spinach, Brussels Sprouts, Purslane, Pastured Eggs/Meat & Dairy Items

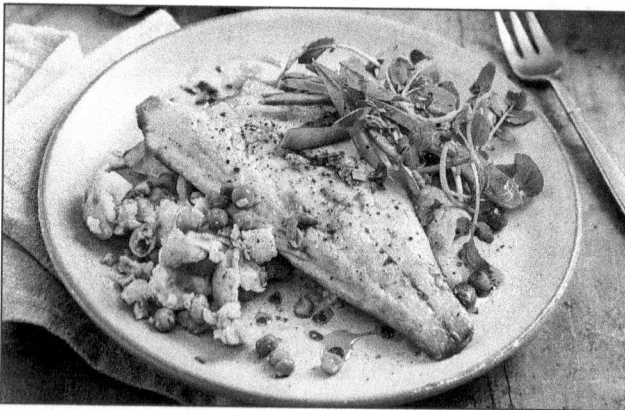

c. <u>Also Present in</u>:

*Forms of Algae, like Chlorella & **Spirulina** [qv. Ingr.#45]*

d. Effect upon Viruses:

Indirectly, by Proper Support of the Immune System *qv.* **e.** Some Reports say EHA & ALA can inhibit Viral Replication

e. Impact on Immunity:

A Healthy Balance of Omega-3 Oils (EPA & DHA) can Decrease Inflammation and Support Immune Functions

f. Additional Information:

Excess Omega-3 Intake Suppresses the Immune System

g. Recommended Daily Intake:

None Provided / Adults – 500 mg per day (Suggested)

h. Human Safety:

Non-Toxic in Suggested Guideline / Food is Safest Source

i. Research Quote - Potential Impact on COVID-19:

"*EPA and DHA* [Omega-3] *supplementation can alter many biological pathways which may have direct influence in the outcome of COVID-19. The safety of EPA and DHA supplementation should be also highlighted. Although, the US Department of Health & Human Services National Institutes of Health Office of Dietary Supplements (ODS) concluded that a daily intake of EPA+DHA of up to 3.0 g/d is safe.*" [20]

j. Research Quote - Recovery from COVID-19:

"*Dietary supplements could possibly improve the patient's recovery. Omega-3 fatty acids, specifically Eicosapentaenoic acid (EPA) and Docosahexaenoic acid (DHA), present an anti-inflammatory effect that could ameliorate some patients need for intensive care unit (ICU) admission. EPA and DHA replace arachidonic acid (ARA) in the phospholipid membranes.* […] *This reduces inflammation.*" [21]

k. Online Dossier of Scientific Research Findings:

https://theantiviraldiet.com/ingredient-%2313-%2B-research

Ingredient #14 ALPHA-LIPOIC ACID

a. Found in:

Spinach, Beef Kidney, Beef Heart, Broccoli, Tomato, Green Peas, Brussels Sprouts, Beef Spleen & Beef Brain

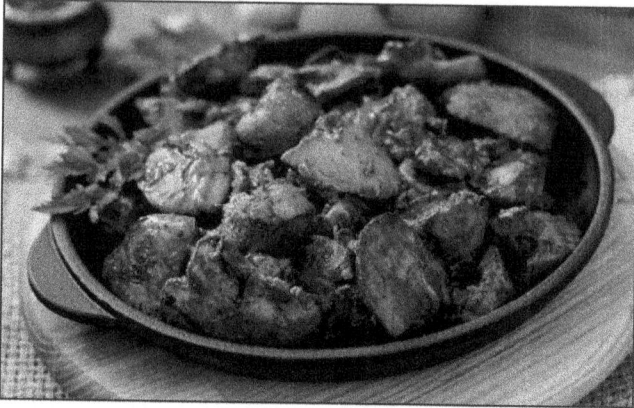

b. Other Sources include:

Rice Bran, Pototoes, Beets, Red Meats (Steaks) & Readily Available in Dietary Supplemention

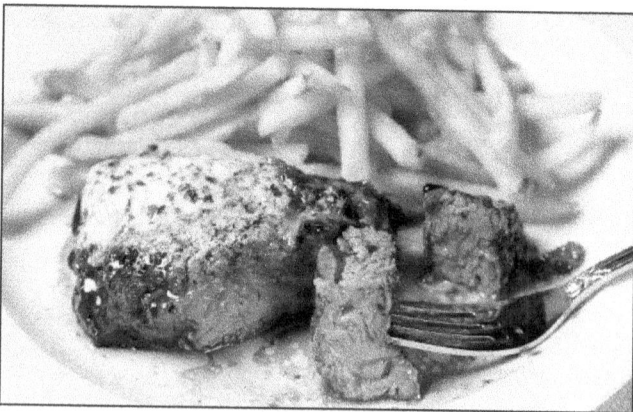

c. Not to be Confused with:

Alpha-Linolenic Acid (as both are abbreviated 'ALA')

d. Effect upon Viruses:
Anti-Viral Action evidenced against Coronavirus 229E, Human Immuno-Deficiency Virus, Vaccinia Virus, Human Influenza A Virus *inter alia*

e. Impact on Immunity:
Positive Effects on both Innate & Adaptive Immune Cells

f. Additional Information:
Regulates the Immune System in Direct and Indirect Ways

g. Recommended Daily Intake:
None Provided / Adults – 200 mg (Suggested Intake)

h. Human Safety:
Check if it interacts with any Medication you are taking

i. Research Quote – Anti-Viral against Coronavirus:
"The addition of a-lipoic acid to G6PD-knockdown cells could attenuate the increased susceptibility to human corona-virus 229E infection. Interestingly, Baur et al. also found that a-lipoic acid was effective to inhibit the replication of HIV-1. In summary, we speculate that ALA could be also used as an optional therapy for this new virus." [2]

j. Research Quote – Effect against COVID-19:
"As the intracellular pH increases, the entry of the virus into the cell decreases. ALA [Alpha Lipoic Acid] can increase human host defense against SARS-CoV-2 by increasing intracellular pH. ALA treatment increases antioxidant levels and reduces oxidative stress. Thus, ALA may strengthen the human host defense against SARS-CoV-2 and can play a vital role in the treatment of patients with critically ill COVID-19." [22]

k. Online Dossier of Scientific Research Findings:
https://theantiviraldiet.com/ingredient-%2314-%2B-research

Ingredient #15 BETA-CAROTENE

a. Found in:

Kale, Spinach, Sweet Potato, Carrots, Broccoli, Butternut Squash, Canteloupe & Red Peppers

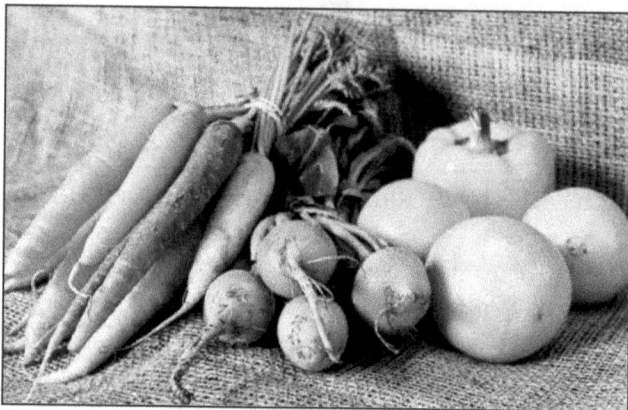

b. Other Sources include:

Yellow Peppers, Apricots, Peas, Romaine Lettuce, Paprika, Cayenne, Chili, Parsley, Sage & Cilantro

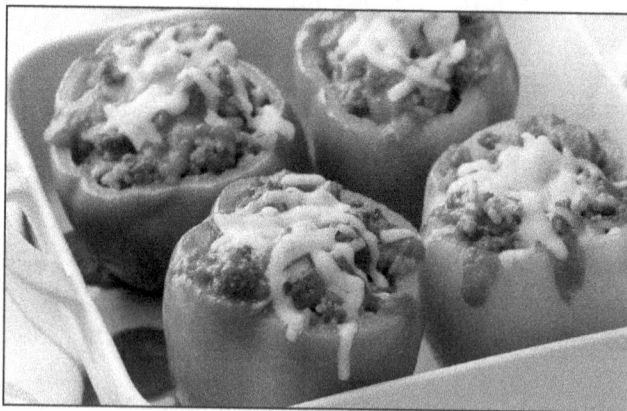

c. Also Known as:

'Pro-Vitamin A' as it converts into Vitamin A [qv. Ingr.#1]

d. Effect upon Viruses:

Anti-Viral Action evidenced against Norovirus, Influenza, Moloney Sarcoma Virus, Poxvirus & Coxsackievirus A16 – due to Positive Impact on levels of Vitamin A in the Body

e. Impact on Immunity:

Increases Immune Cells *incl.* CD4 & Natural Killer Cells

f. Additional Information:

Stops Breakdown of Cells & Tissues caused by Oxidation

g. Recommended Daily Intake:

Adults – 4.8 mg per day (for 800 mcg of Vitamin A)

h. Human Safety:

Non-Toxic within RDI Guidelines / Food is Safest Source

i. Research Quote – Immuno-Modulatory Effect:

"The action of carotenoids on immune response hangs in a delicate balance with the intra- and extra-cellular milieu, the outcome of which depends not only on the type and concentration of the carotenoid but also on the cell type and animal species involved. Even though studies to date have provided evidence for a specific action of carotenoids, much has yet to be done to truly understand their molecular action." [23]

j. Research Quote – Effect upon SARS-CoV-2:

"β-Carotene and other carotenoids have been reported to possess immunomodulatory activities in humans and animals. These carotenoids enhance lymphocyte blastogenesis, increase the population of specific lymphocyte subsets, increase lymphocyte cytotoxic activity, and stimulate the production of various cytokines." [24]

k. Online Dossier of Scientific Research Findings:

https://theantiviraldiet.com/ingredient-%2315-%2B-research

Ingredient #16 BETA GLUCANS

a. Found in:

Barley Fibre, Oats, Whole Grains (Millet, Quinoa, Bulgur, Barley), Wild Rice, Shiitake & Brown Rice

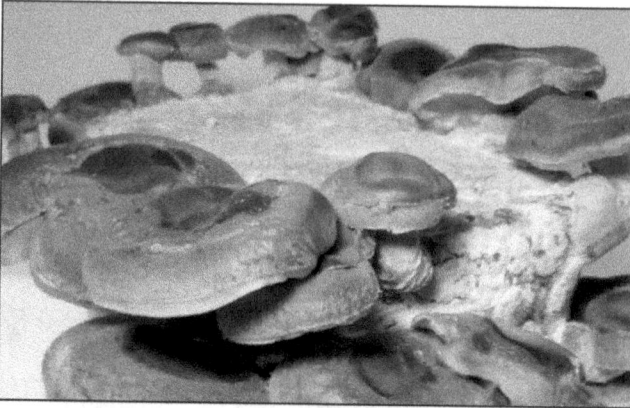

b. Other Sources include:

Other Whole Grains (Popcorn, Whole Rye, Buckwheat Wheat Berry, Freekeh, Sorghum), Seaweed & Algae

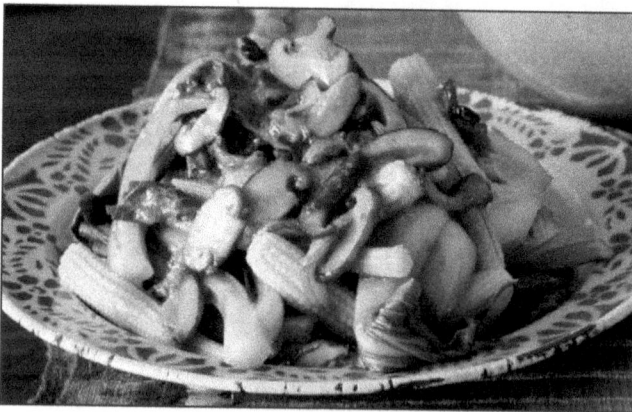

c. Also Found in:

Maitake and Reishi Mushrooms [qv. Ingrs.#47 & #48]

d. Effect upon Viruses:
Indirectly, by Stimulation of the Immune System qv. **e.**

e. Impact on Immunity:
Increases Immune Response by activating Complement System, improving Macrophages and Natural Killer Cell Functioning. Innate & Adaptive Immunity are Increased

f. Additional Information:
Also ameliorates Cholesterol Levels and Heart Health

g. Recommended Daily Intake:
None Provided / Intake Recommended During an Illness

h. Human Safety:
Check if it interacts with any Medication you are taking

i. Research Quote - Therapeutic for COVID-19:
"Our findings demonstrate significant physicochemical differences between Lentinan [β-Glucan] extracts, which produce differential in vitro immunomodulatory and pulmonary cytoprotective effects that may also have positive relevance to candidate COVID-19 therapeutics targeting cytokine storm." [25]

j. Research Quote - Phytotherapy against COVID-19:
"The extracts described in this review [including β-Glucans] have been proven to possess great antiviral activities, with a general consensus of low toxicity. In addition, compared to commercial pharmaceuticals, such medicinal herbs are readily available and much cheaper. With the current pandemic, many scientists have rushed to the development of a potential vaccine and therapeutic agent that is effective against COVID-19; however, herbal agents should not be overlooked." [26]

k. Online Dossier of Scientific Research Findings:
https://theantiviraldiet.com/ingredient-%2316-%2B-research

Ingredient #17 L-CARNITINE

a. <u>Found in</u>:

Red Meat (above all Beef Steak), Ground Beef, Codfish, Grilled Chicken, Smoked Meat & Tuna

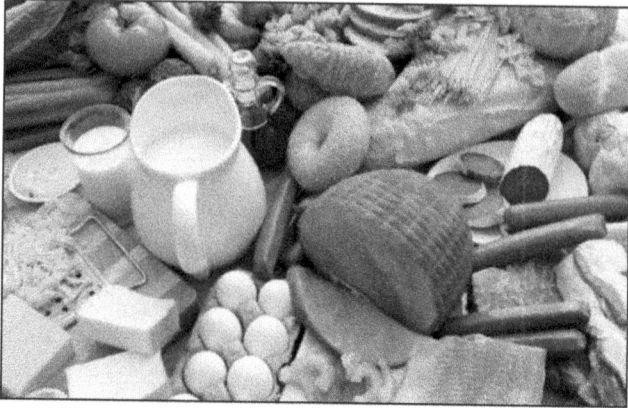

b. <u>Other Sources include</u>:

Milk, Ice-Cream, Cheese, Eggs, Wholewheat Bread, Avocado, Spinach, Asparagus, Beans & Chickpeas

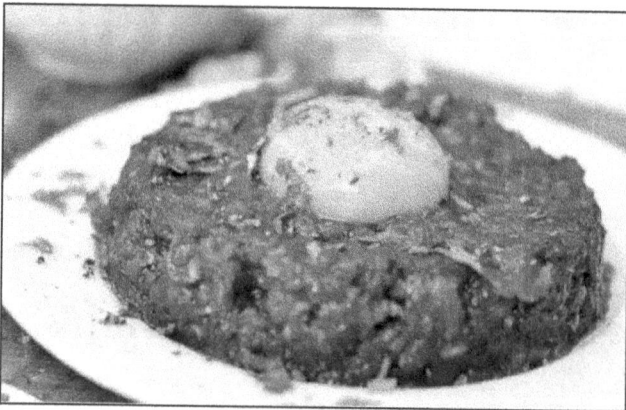

c. <u>Observation</u>:

Vegetarian Diets are naturally low in nutrient L-Carnitine

d. Effect upon Viruses:
Anti-Viral Action evidenced against Hepatitis C, Dengue Fever Virus Type 2, Influenza A Virus (H5N1) *inter alia*

e. Impact on Immunity:
Increases the Proliferation of T-Lymphocytes, improving function of Neutrophils. Improves Immunity in the Elderly

f. Additional Information:
Some Evidence it reduces Fatigue & limits Muscle Damage

g. Recommended Daily Intake:
None Given / Adults – 500 mg per day (Suggested)

h. Human Safety:
Non-Toxic in Suggested Guideline / Food is Safest Source

i. Research Quote – Potential against COVID-19:
"[I]t is expected that the supplementation of patients with L-Carnitine in primary stages of the disease [COVID-19] could prevent the deterioration of overall health and the fatal complications of the virus." [27]

j. Research Quote – Immuno-Modulatory Effects:
"The results showed that T cell function increased in patients treated with ALC [L-Carnitine], but decreased in patients receiving placebo. The immunomodulatory effect of ALC could be attributed to: (1) its ability to supplement energy needed by lymphocytes to fight infection; (2) its ability to prevent chemotherapeutic impairment of lymphocyte function or potentiate lymphocyte antibacterial activity; and (3) the release of immuno-enhancing neurohormones and neuropeptides through its ability to modulate the hypothalamus-pituitary-adrenal axis." [28]

k. Online Dossier of Scientific Research Findings:
https://theantiviraldiet.com/ingredient-%2317-%2B-research

FLAVONOIDS

FLAVONOIDS, A CLASS of plant Polyphenols, are a type of biochemical pigment that were found to be of massive benefits to human health during the twentieth century. They were first discovered by the Hungarian biochemist Albert Szent-Gyorgyi in 1937, who went on to win a Nobel prize for his research on Bioflavonoids and Vitamin C. - Also known as the Flavones, this group of chemicals appears in many plants and is responsible for a number of the colours that we see in flowers, leaves and fruit. For instance, one group of flavonoids, called the 'Anthocyanins', are the main chemical responsible for giving a purple-red colour to Autumn leaves - and also the red colouring typical in buds and small shoots. Another group of flavonoids called the 'Anthoxanthins' give a yellow colour to the petals of numerous flowers. Why these chemicals impart the colours that they do, is not known for definite, though it is possible that the pigmentation they give to plants exerts a power of attraction on bees and butterflies. In that way, these and other pollen-transporting creatures are encouraged towards these plants, causing them to bring about fertilization. Plant Polyphenols, as far as humans are concerned, are micronutrients with antioxidant properties and have many health benefits. They appear to successfully treat digestion issues, to assist with weight management and also to alleviate diabetes, cardiovascular diseases, even neurodegenerative conditions.

In this sub-section are included six ingredients that belong to this class of naturally occurring compounds. Just a few words of introduction are given to them here, without delving into their key anti-viral and immunomodulatory properties.

Quercetin, one of the best researched flavonoids, has significant antioxidant effects, eliminating unstable molecules and thus preventing cellular damage. Evidence exists that the decrease in 'Free Radical' molecules can help us avoid cancer, diabetes and heart disease. Quercetin is one of the most common flavonoids in our diets, for it is found in a wide variety of food - including apples, onions, broccoli, chocolate and wine.

Naringenin is another widely occurring flavonoid as it is present in a number of citrus fruits, tomatoes and bergamot. Like Quercetin, research has evidenced it to have antioxidant properties, to fight inflammation and even have inhibitory effects upon cancers and tumour growth. Further studies are being undertaken on its bioavailability and cardioprotectivity.

Hesperidin, like Naringenin, is found in citrus fruits - though across an even wider number of them. It was first discovered in 1828 by French chemist Lebreton and it is highly prized for some of its medicinal effects. Evidence shows that Hesperidin is beneficial to blood circulation - being effective treatment for hemorrhoids, varicose veins and venous stasis.

Apigenin, present in many fruits and vegetables, is especially found in celery, parsley and celeriac. This flavonoid has evidence supporting its benefits against diabetes, amnesia, depression, insomnia, cancer and neurodegeneration. It appears to be most abundantly found in chamomile leaves.

Rutin, for a couple of decades acclaimed as Vitamin P (mid-1930s to early 1950s), is a well-researched flavonoid in terms of its biochemical reactions and therapeutic potential. It is a citrus flavonoid though also present in plums, peaches, buckwheat and asparagus. Like the others above, it has shown antioxidant, anti-inflammatory and anticancer properties.

EGCG, or *Epigallo-Catechin-3-Gallate*, is the flavonoid most abundantly found in Green Tea, though present in smaller quantities in White Tea and Black Tea. It has been extensively studied and a significant body of research attests to its anti-cancer, anti-bacterial and high antioxidant qualities.

There are many other important flavonoids, some of which will also deserve a place in this diet but for which more research is being undertaken before they can be included. Other significant flavonoids to mention too, are Morin, Taxifolin, Herbacetin, Luteolin, Quercetrin, Cinanserin and Fisetin.

Ingredient #18 QUERCETIN

a. Found in:

Dockleaf, Watercress, Cilantro, Radicchio, Asparagus, Okra, Elderberry, Blueberry, Blackberry, Fig & Apples

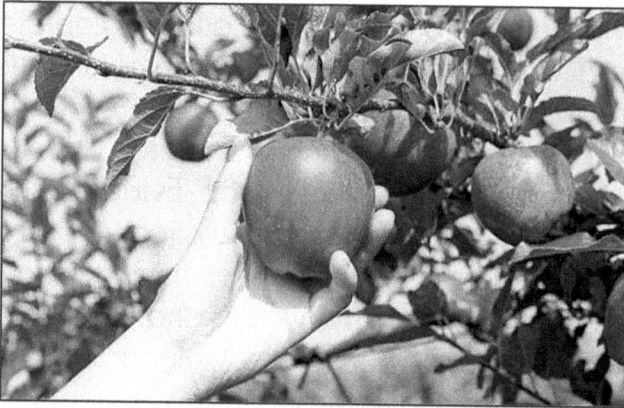

b. Other Sources include:

Serrano Peppers, Red Onion, Redleaf Lettuce, Broccoli, Kale, Mulberry, Grapes, Green Tea, Coffee & Capers

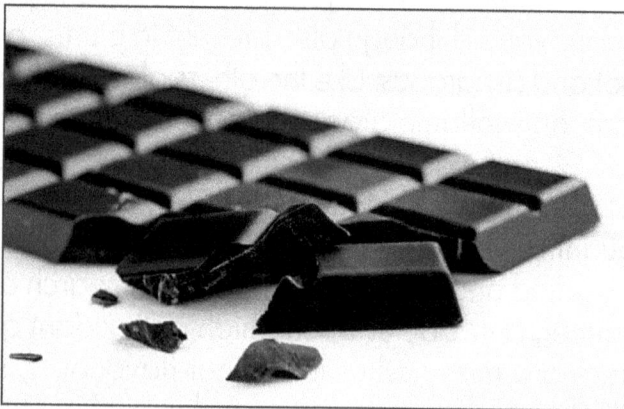

c. Also Found in:

Dark Chocolate (as it is in Cocoa Beans) and Red Wine

d. Effect upon Viruses:
Anti-Viral Action evidenced against SARS-CoV-1, Herpes Simplex Virus Type 1, (HSV-1), Poliovirus Type 1, Para-influenza Virus Type 3 (PF3), Respiratory Syncytial Virus (RSV), Influenza A Virus (IAV), Hepatitis C Virus, Ebola Virus, Zika Virus, Enterovirus-71, MERS-CoV *inter alia*

e. Impact on Immunity:
Main Impact of Quercetin is Direct Anti-Viral Action *qv.* **d.**

f. Additional Information:
It is a Powerful Antioxidant and Inhibits Histamine Release

g. Recommended Daily Intake: Not Applicable

h. Human Safety: Non-Toxic but Excess may be harmful

i. Research Quote - Potential Use against COVID-19:
"It's known that COVID-19 goes with excessive immune reaction of human body in severe cases. Quercetin is reported to be effective on treatment and prophylaxis of other SARS like coronavirus infections, as a strong antioxidant and scavenger flavonoid without any adverse events. Upon this data, the investigators hypothesize that quercetin can be effective on both prophylaxis and treatment of COVID-19 cases." [29]

j. Research Quote - Anti-Viral/Immuno-Modulatory:
"Quercetin displays a broad range of antiviral properties which can interfere at multiple steps of pathogen virulence - virus entry, virus replication, protein assembly." [4]

"Quercetin exhibits both immunomodulatory and anti-microbial effects in preclinical studies. [...] One study reported a decrease in incidence of upper respiratory tract infection." [30]

k. Online Dossier of Scientific Research Findings:
https://theantiviraldiet.com/ingredient-%2318-%2B-research

Ingredient #19 NARINGENIN

a. Found in:

Pummelo, Grapefruits, Tangerines, Oranges, Grapes, Greek Oregano, Almonds & Pistacchios

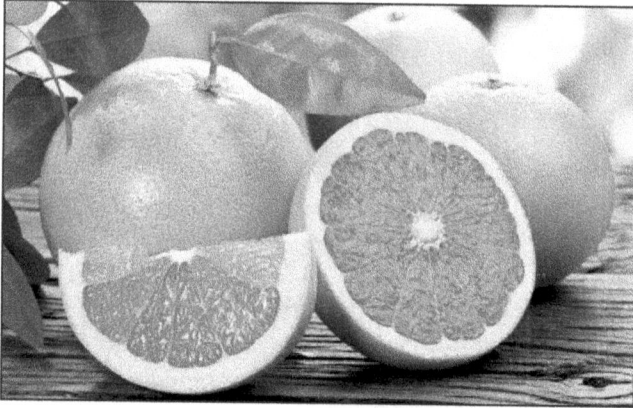

b. Other Sources include:

Limes, Lemons, Bergamot, Sour Orange, Tomatoes, Tart Cherries, Water Mint, Cocoa & Red Wine

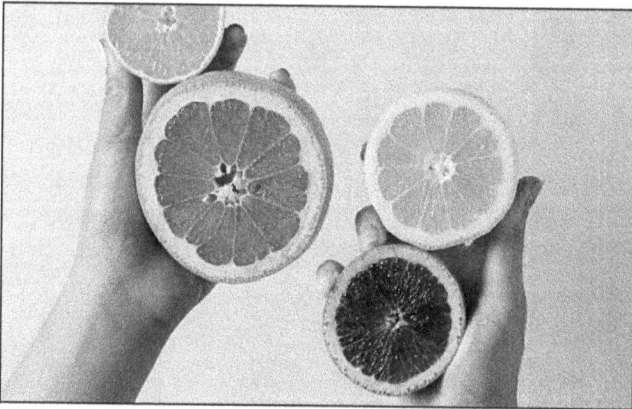

c. Observation:

Naringenin itself is both Colourless and Flavourless

d. Effect upon Viruses:
Anti-Viral Action evidenced against Herpes Simplex Virus (HSV-1), Dengue Fever Virus Type-2, Canine Distemper Virus, Zika Virus, Hepatitis C Virus & Chikungunya Virus

e. Impact on Immunity:
Main Impact of Naringenin is Direct Anti-Viral Action *qv.* d. It modulates Immune Response to manage Inflammation

f. Additional Information:
It is a Powerful Antioxidant and has Bactericidal Effects

g. Recommended Daily Intake: Not Applicable

h. Human Safety: Non-Toxic but Excess may be harmful

i. Research Quote – Anti-Viral against SARS-CoV-2:
"In conclusion, these considerations offer a perspective on specific molecular targets, TPCs, and underpin a role for Naringenin as pharmacological blockade of SARS-CoV-2 infectivity providing further support for exploration of TPCs inhibition as novel antiviral therapy." [31]

j. Research Quote – Potential against COVID-19:
"The evidence reviewed here indicates that naringenin might exert therapeutic effects against COVID-19 through the inhibition of COVID-19 main protease, 3-chymotrypsin-like protease (3CLpro), and reduction of angiotensin converting enzyme receptors activity. One of the other mechanisms by which naringenin might exert therapeutic effects against COVID-19 is, at least partly, by attenuating inflammatory responses. The anti-viral activity of the flavanone naringenin against some viruses has also been reported. On the whole, the favorable effects of naringenin lead to a conclusion that naringenin may be a promising treatment strategy against COVID-19." [32]

k. Online Dossier of Scientific Research Findings:
https://theantiviraldiet.com/ingredient-%2319-%2B-research

Ingredient #20 HESPERIDIN

a. Found in:

*Oranges, Tangerines, Lemons, Limes, Grapefruit,
Sun-Dried Tangerine Peels & Peppermint*

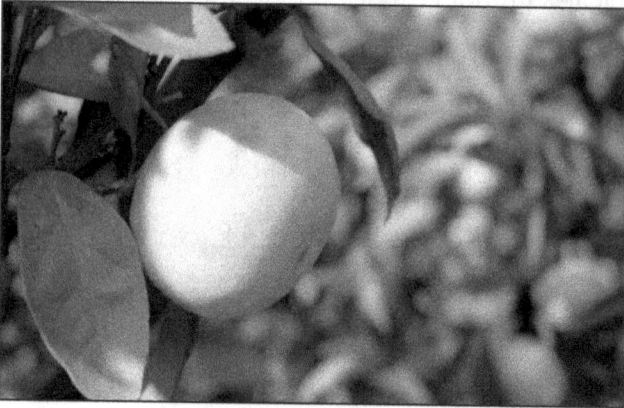

b. Other Sources include:

*Several Herbs, incl. Ramie, Dangshen, Nanche,
Japanese Catnip, Indian Valerian & Honeybush*

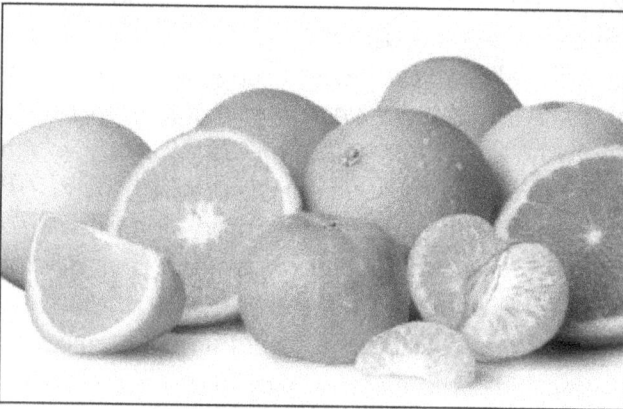

c. Highest Content:

Peppermint is Most Concentrated Source of Hesperidin

d. Effect upon Viruses:

Anti-Viral Action evidenced against Rotavirus, Influenza A Virus, Zika Virus, Chikungunya Virus (CHIKV) *inter alia*

e. Impact on Immunity:

Main Impact of Hesperidin is Direct Anti-Viral Action *qv.* **d.** It modulates Immune Response to manage Inflammation

f. Additional Information:

Hesperidin improves the Self-Renewal Ability of Tissues. It has Antioxidant, Antibacterial & Anti-Allergic Effects. It is currently being researched **re:** SARS-CoV-2 Virus

g. Recommended Daily Intake: Not Applicable

h. Human Safety: Non-Toxic but Excess may be harmful

i. Research Quote - Anti-Viral/Immuno-Modulatory:

"*Anti-viral activity of hesperidin might constitute a treatment option for COVID-19 through improving host cellular immunity against infection and its good anti-inflammatory activity may help in controlling cytokine storm. Hesperidin mixture with diosmin co-administrated with heparin protect against venous thromboembolism which may prevent disease progression. Based on that, hesperidin might be used as a meaningful pro-phylactic agent and a promising adjuvant treatment option against SARS-CoV-2 infection.*" [33]

j. Research Quote - Anti-Viral against SARS-CoV-2:

"*Among the latter, hesperidin has recently attracted the atten-tion of researchers, because it binds to the key proteins of the SARS-CoV-2 virus [...]. The affinity of hesperidin for these pro-teins is comparable if not superior to that of common chemi-cal antivirals.*" [34]

k. Online Dossier of Scientific Research Findings:

https://theantiviraldiet.com/ingredient-%2320-%2B-research

Ingredient #21 APIGENIN

a. Found in:

Grapefruit, Onions, Oranges, Artichoke, Parsley, Celery, Tea, Chamomile, Wheat Sprouts & Wine

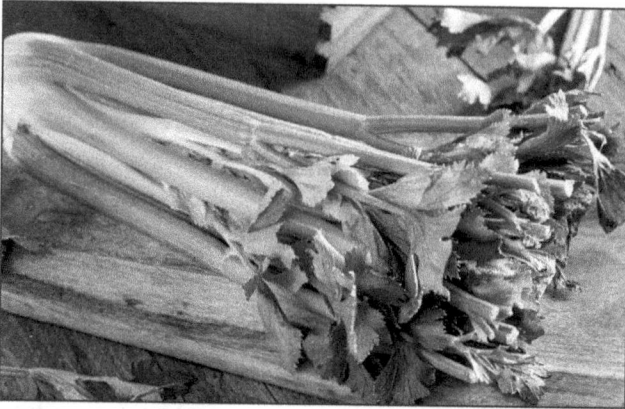

b. Other Sources include:

Rutabagas, Thyme, Iceberg Lettuce & Celeriac

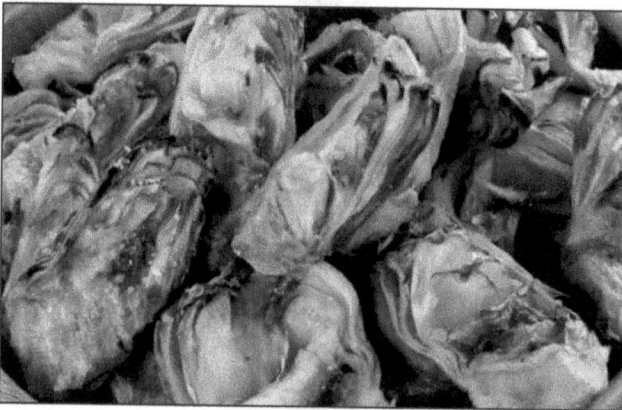

c. Also Found in:

Beer - above all when brewed with Natural Ingredients

d. Effect upon Viruses:
Anti-Viral Action evidenced against Enterovirus-71, Epstein-Barr Virus, Herpes Simplex Virus Type 1, Herpes Simplex Virus Type 2, Hepatitis C Virus, Influenza Virus *inter alia*

e. Impact on Immunity:
Main Impact of Apigenin is Direct Anti-Viral Action *qv.* d.

f. Additional Information:
Also Anti-Inflammatory, Antioxidant and Bactericidal. It is currently being researched **re:** SARS-CoV-2 Virus

g. Recommended Daily Intake: Not Applicable

h. Human Safety: Non-Toxic but Excess may be harmful

i. Research Quote – Anti-Viral against SARS-CoV-2:
"*Fisetin, quercetin, isorhamnetin, genistein, luteolin, resveratrol and* **apigenin** *on the other hand, interact with the S2 domain of spike protein with the binding energies of -8.5, -8.5, -8.3, -8.2, -8.2, -7.9, -7.7 Kcal/mol, respectively. Our study suggested that, these flavonoid and non-flavonoid moieties have significantly high binding affinity for the two main important domains of the spike protein which is responsible for the attachment and internalization of the virus in the host cell and their binding affinities are much higher compared to that of HCQ* [Hydroxychloroquine]." [35]

j. Research Quote – Anti-Viral Flavonoid Action:
"*Apigenin has been associated with antiviral effects, together with quercetin, rutin, and other flavonoids. The antiviral activity appears to be connected to the non-glycosidic compounds, and hydroxylation at the 3-position is apparently a prerequisite for antiviral activity.*" [36]

k. Online Dossier of Scientific Research Findings:
https://theantiviraldiet.com/ingredient-%2321-%2B-research

Ingredient #22 RUTIN

a. <u>Found in</u>:

Capers (spice) Buckwheat, Cherries, Olives, Plums, Grapefruit, Greencurrant, Apples & Passion Flower

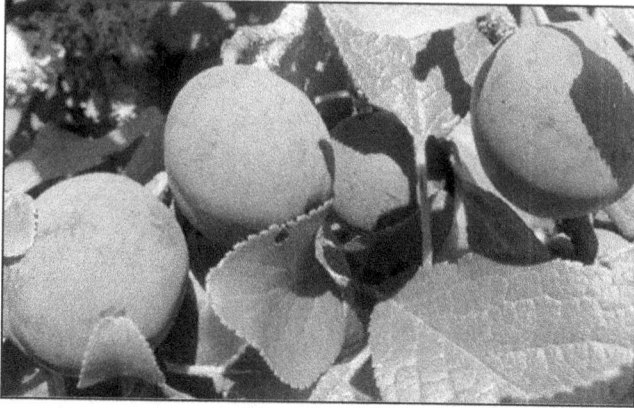

b. <u>Other Sources include</u>:

Asparagus, Raspberries, Buckwheat Groats, Apricots, Prune, Cherry Tomato, Fenugreek, Marjoram & Zucchini

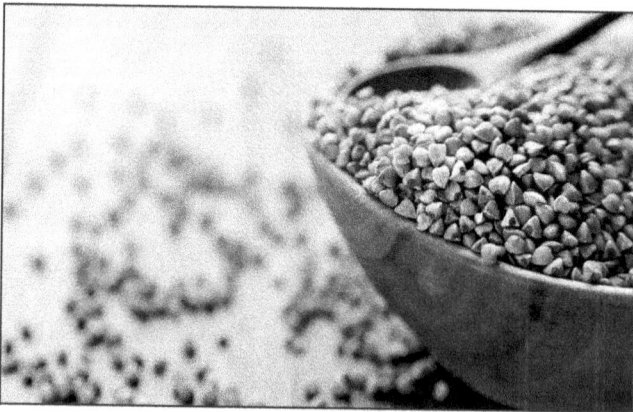

c. <u>Also Found in</u>:

Green Tea and Black Tea (although in Small Quantities)

d. Effect upon Viruses:
Anti-Viral Action evidenced against Influenza Virus, Dengue Fever Virus Type 2, Hepatitis C Virus & Enterovirus A71

e. Impact on Immunity:
Main Impact of Rutin is via Direct Anti-Viral Action *qv.* d.

f. Additional Information:
Also Anti-Inflammatory, Antioxidant and Bactericidal. Rutin was originally known as 'Vitamin P' or 'Rutoside'. It is currently being researched **re:** SARS-CoV-2 Virus

g. Recommended Daily Intake: Not Applicable

h. Human Safety: Non-Toxic but Excess may be harmful

i. Research Quote – Anti-Viral against SARS-CoV-2:
"It is well known that the main protease (Mpro) of SARS-CoV-2 plays an important role in maturation of many viral proteins such as the RNA-dependent RNA polymerase. Here, we explore the underlying molecular mechanisms of the computationally determined top candidate – rutin, a key component in many traditional antiviral medicines such as Lianhuaqinwen and Shuanghuanlian, for inhibiting the viral target–Mpro." [37]

j. Research Quote – Potential against Coronaviruses:
"The citrus flavonoid rutin was identified to fit snugly into the Mpro substrate-binding pocket and to present a strong interaction with TLRs TLR2, TLR6 and TLR7. One-carbon metabolic process and nitrogen metabolism ranked high as potential targets toward rutin. Conclusion: Rutin may influence viral functional protein assembly and host inflammatory suppression. Its affinity for Mpro and TLRs render rutin a potential novel therapeutic anti-coronavirus strategy." [38]

k. Online Dossier of Scientific Research Findings:
https://theantiviraldiet.com/ingredient-%2322-%2B-research

Ingredient #23 EGCG

Epigallo-Catechin-3-Gallate

a. Found in:

Green Tea, White Tea, Oolong & Black Teas

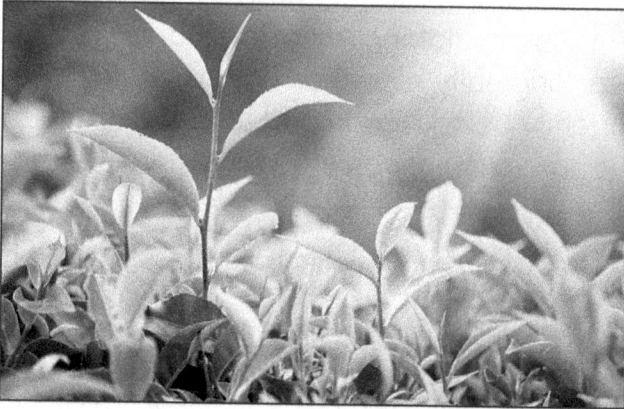

b. Other Sources include:

Cranberries, Cherries, Pears, Peaches, Apples, Kiwis, Strawberries, Avocados & Blackberries

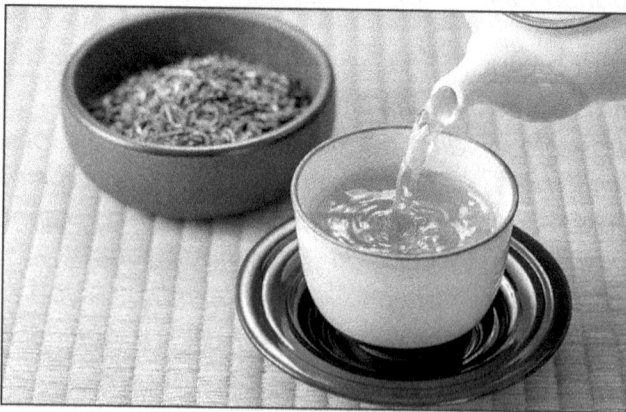

c. Also Found in:

Some Nuts - such as Pecans, Pistachios and Hazelnuts

d. Effect upon Viruses:

Anti-Viral Action evidenced against Human Immunodeficiency Virus, Influenza A Virus, Rotavirus, Hepatitis B Virus, Hepatitis C Virus, Adenovirus, Epstein-Barr Virus, Enterovirus-71, Human Norovirus, Chikungunya Virus *inter alia*

e. Impact on Immunity:

Main Impact of EGCG is via Direct Anti-Viral Action *qv.* d.

f. Additional Information:

Also Anti-Inflammatory, Antioxidant and Bactericidal.

g. Recommended Daily Intake: Not Applicable

h. Human Safety: Non-Toxic but Excess can be harmful

i. Research Quote - Potential against COVID-19:

"*Altogether, our findings reveal that green tea catechins/ polyphenols (especially EGCG, ECG and GCG) can be potent anti-COVID-19 drug candidates. Additionally, this study opens up futuristic testing (in vitro and in vivo) possibilities of these three green tea polyphenols against COVID-19.*" [39]

j. Research Quote - Anti-Viral for SARS-CoV-2 *et al*:

"*Recent studies have revealed the possible binding sites present on SARS-CoV-2 and studied their interactions with tea polyphenols. EGCG and theaflavins, especially theaflavin-3,3'-digallate (TF3) have shown a significant interaction with the receptors under consideration in this review. Some docking studies further emphasize on the activity of these polyphenols against COVID-19.*" [40]

"*Further studies are required to understand the exact mechanism of viral inhibition [...] spirulina and green tea could be promising antiviral agents against emerging viruses.*" [41]

k. Online Dossier of Scientific Research Findings:

https://theantiviraldiet.com/ingredient-%2323-%2B-research

HERBS & SPICES

UNLIKE THE FOUR PREVIOUS sub-sections - where each of the ingredients given an entry was one specific chemical or group of chemicals - in this and the following two sub-sections *some* of the ingredients are referred to by their chemical names, while *others* are given the names by which they are more commonly known. In the case of herbs and spices within this section, though it may be less scientific to call a herb by its traditional name, the effectiveness of some of these ingredients appears to be due to the combination of chemicals in them and not due to a single compound alone. The last four entries in this section should properly be called *herbs* as they are derived from the herbaceous (or 'grassy') part of a plant, whereas the first five ingredients are *spices* as they are generally taken from other parts of the plant - often dessicated - including the seeds, the bark, fruits and roots. Ingredients from these parts of the plant are sometimes evidenced to have higher efficacy for health purposes when still in fresh form *e.g.* ginger. A few words of introduction on the general nature of the herbs and spices will describe some of their key qualities.

Allicin is the name of the active ingredient found in the highest quantity in Garlic (*Allium Sativum*). It was only produced synthetically by Chester J. Cavallito and John Hays Bailey in 1944. Accounts of its ability to treat and cure illness go back to antiquity. It has proven anti-bacterial, anti-fungal, anti-parasitic, anti-inflammatory and anti-viral properties.

Galangal, in its four main forms, is a 'Rhizome', a plant with numerous creeping stems and rootstalks. These are used fresh or dried out for later use. Traditionally, Galangal has been taken for alleviating stomach and digestion problems, as well as for treating respiratory diseases. It is a known anti-inflammatory.

Curcumin is the main bioactive component within the Indian spice Turmeric, from which it receives its bright orange colour. It has been extensively studied and appears to have some anti-inflammatory, antioxidant and anti-cancer qualities – among others – but low bioavailability is an issue of concern.

Ginger is one of the best known spices and contains a number of powerful chemicals, including '6-Gingerol', which simulated molecular docking shows may be a promising medicine for COVID-19. Ginger is also a known anti-inflammatory.

Piperine is an alkaloid, known for its effect on humans, which is found in many forms of pepper, above all black pepper. It is known for its numerous health benefits, including reduction of insulin resistance and as being anti-inflammatory.

Rosemary, containing Rosmarinic Acid and other bioactive compounds, has potent antioxidant effects as well as being an anti-inflammatory and improving blood circulation.

Oregano, also known as 'Sweet Marjoram' is a staple herb in Italian cuisine. It is high in antioxidants, has anti-bacterial properties and evidence also shows it may fight cancer.

Sage, also known as 'Salvia Officinalis', is a widely-used herb in many countries. In the Levant and Egypt it is also a popular tea infusion. It is high in nutrients and antioxidants.

Peppermint, one of the most popular herbs – used in a condiment for Roast Lamb, as tea, in flavourings for chocolate, sweets *etc.* – is also anti-bacterial and soothes indigestion.

As for *Basil*, the popular herb used in Pesto, it also has serious anti-oxidant, anti-inflammatory qualities. In recent years, *Holy Basil* (Tulsi) has been shown to have anti-bacterial, anti-fungal, anti-inflammatory and analgesic properties.

There were several other herbs and spices which may be deserving of inclusion in such an anti-viral diet, however – as was the case in previous sections – the test has always been whether enough scientific evidence currently exists to merit the presence of a specific dietary element. Science remains throughout the test for inclusion or exclusion of an ingredient. Capsaicin, for example, does have *some* evidence in favour of its anti-viral capacity – even in terms of SARS-CoV-2 – but additional results and corroboration are still being awaited.

Ingredient #24 ALLICIN

a. Found in:
Garlic, Onions, Shallots, Chinese Chives & Leeks

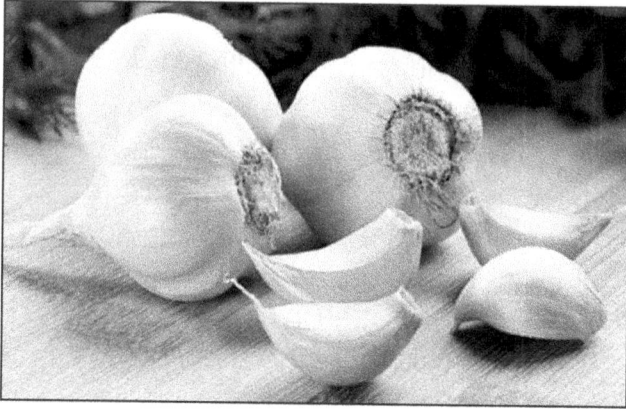

b. Also Found in:
Garlic Paste, Garlic Oil, Garlic Butter & Garlic Pepper

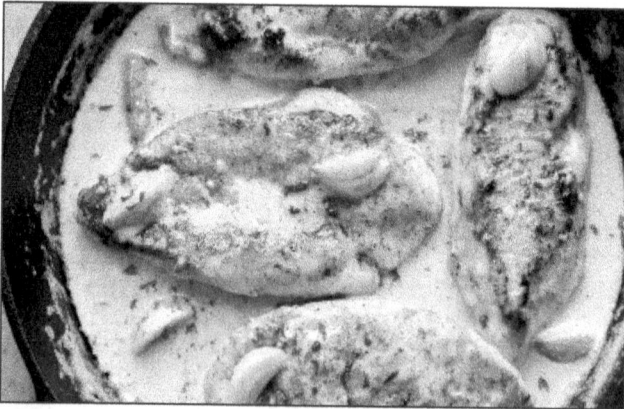

c. Historically:
Garlic is well documented as having been used by the Egyptians, Babylonians, Greeks, Romans and Chinese

d. Effect upon Viruses:
Anti-Viral Action evidenced against Influenzas, Infectious Bronchitis Virus, Herpes Simplex Virus Type 1, Herpes Simplex Virus Type 2, Dengue Fever Virus, Parainfluenza Virus Type 3, Vaccinia Virus, Vesicular Stomatitis Virus, Human Rhinovirus Type 2 & Cytomegalovirus Virus

e. Impact on Immunity:
Main Impact of Allicin is via Direct Anti-Viral Action qv. d.

f. Additional Information:
When Garlic is sliced, crushed or chewed the Compound 'Alliin' chemically converts into Active Ingredient 'Allicin'

g. Recommended Daily Intake: Not Applicable

h. Human Safety: Non-Toxic but Excess can be harmful

i. Research Quote – Anti-Viral against SARS-CoV-2:
"*The results suggest that the garlic essential oil is a valuable natural antivirus source, which contributes to preventing the invasion of coronavirus into the human body.*" [42]

"*The results suggested that alliin may serve as a good candidate as an inhibitor of SARS-CoV-2 Mpro. Therefore, the present research may provide some meaningful guidance for the prevention and treatment of SARS-CoV-2.*" [43]

j. Research Quote – Potential against COVID-19:
"*In conclusion, Allium sativum may be an acceptable preventive measure against COVID-19 infection to boost immune system cells and to repress the production and secretion of proinflammatory cytokines as well as an adipose tissue derived hormone leptin having the proinflammatory nature.*" [44]

k. Online Dossier of Scientific Research Findings:
https://theantiviraldiet.com/ingredient-%2324-%2B-research

Ingredient #25 GALANGAL

a. <u>Found in 2 Main Forms:</u>

*Both as **Alpinia Galanga** ('Greater Galangal')
and as **Alpinia Officinarum** ('Lesser Galangal')*

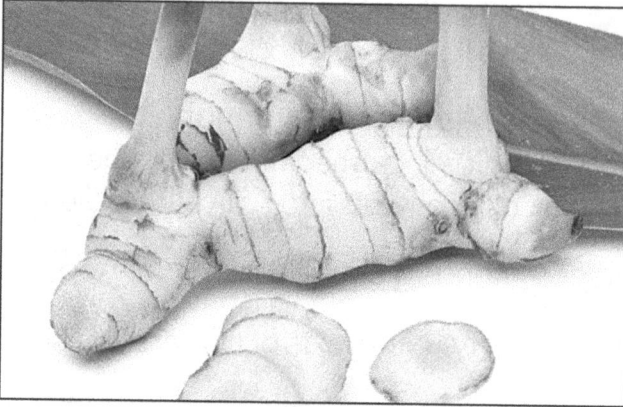

b. <u>Other Forms of Galangal are:</u>

Boesenbergia Rotunda *('Chinese Ginger' or 'Finger Root')*
Kaempferia Galanga *('Black Galangal' or 'Sand Ginger')*

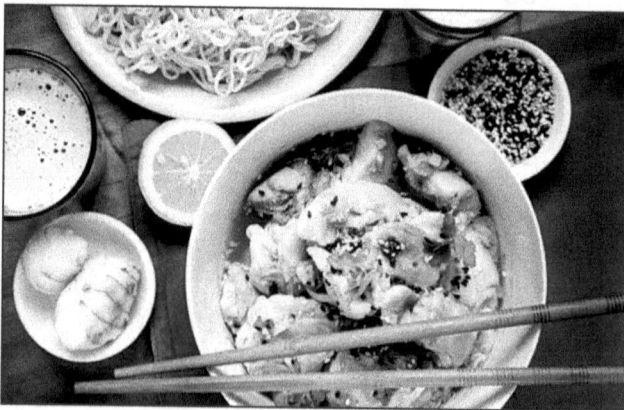

c. <u>Please Note that:</u>

Anti-Viral Effects only shown in Greater/Lesser Galangal

d. Effect upon Viruses:
Anti-Viral Action evidenced against Respiratory Syncytial Virus, Poliovirus, Measles Virus, Herpes Simplex Virus Type 1, Influenza Virus, Human Immunodeficiency Virus *inter alia*

e. Impact on Immunity:
Main Impact of Bioactive Ingredients of Galangal [by Galangin *et alia*] is via Direct Anti-Viral Action *qv.* **d.**

f. Additional Information:
It is currently being researched **re:** SARS-CoV-2 Virus

g. Recommended Daily Intake: Not Applicable

h. Human Safety: Non-Toxic but Excess may be harmful

i. Research Quote – Protection against COVID-19:
"In general, the results of this study indicate that Citrus sp. exhibit the best potential as an inhibitor to the development of the SARS-CoV-2, followed by Galangal, Sappan wood, and Curcuma sp. that can be consumed in daily life as prophylaxis of COVID-19." [45]

j. Research Quote – Anti-Viral against SARS-CoV-2:
"We prepared an in house library of compounds found in rhizomes, Alpinia officinarum, ginger and curcuma, and docked them into the solvent accessible S3–S4 pocket of PLpro. Eight compounds from Alpinia officinarum and ginger bind with high in silico affinity to closed PLpro conformer, and hence are potential SARS-CoV-2 PLpro inhibitors. Our study reveal new lead compounds targeting SARS-CoV-2. Further structure based modifications or extract formulations of these compounds can lead to highly potent inhibitors to treat SARS-CoV-2 infections." [46]

k. Online Dossier of Scientific Research Findings:
https://theantiviraldiet.com/ingredient-%2325-%2B-research

Ingredient #26 CURCUMIN

a. Found as:

*Principle Curcuminoid in **Turmeric** (Curcuma Longa) - one member of the Ginger family, Zingiberaceae*

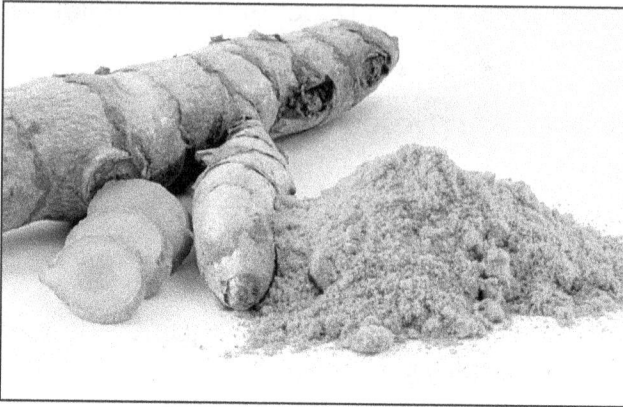

b. Widely Used as:

Powdered Turmeric, one of the main Indian Spices - identifiable by its signature yellow-orange colour

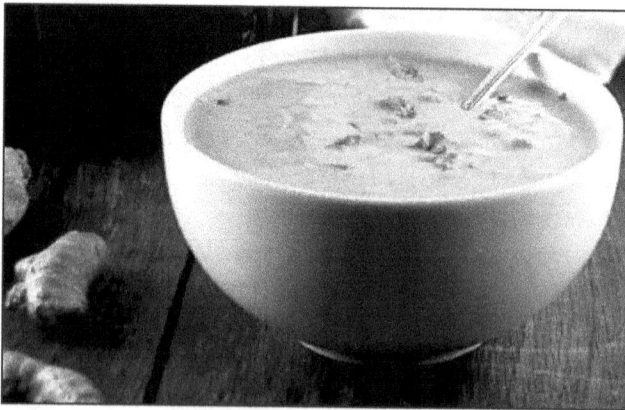

c. Ayurvedic Use:

Turmeric was used to Decrease all sorts of Inflammation

d. Effect upon Viruses:

Anti-Viral Action evidenced against Zika Virus, Chikungunya Virus, Herpes Simplex Virus Type 1, Respiratory Syncytial Virus, Enteric Coronavirus, Human Immunodeficiency Virus (HIV-1), Hepatitis B Virus, Hepatitis C Virus, Coxsackievirus B3, Influenza A Virus *inter alia*

e. Impact on Immunity:

Main Impact of Curcumin is Direct Anti-Viral Action *qv.* d.

f. Additional Information:

Also Anti-Inflammatory, Antioxidant and Bactericidal. It is currently being researched **re:** SARS-CoV-2 Virus

g. Recommended Daily Intake: Not Applicable

h. Human Safety: Non-Toxic but Excess may be harmful

i. Research Quote - Anti-Viral against SARS-CoV-2:

"A good binding energy, drug likeness and efficient pharmacokinetic parameters suggest the potential of curcumin and a few of its derivatives as SARS-CoV-2 spike protein inhibitors. However, further research is necessary to investigate the ability of these compounds as viral entry inhibitors." [47]

j. Research Quote - Prevention against COVID-19:

"Henceforth, it is clear that the biological properties including advance mode of drug delivery system of curcumin could be considered while formulating the pharmaceutical products and its application as preventive measure in the inhibition of transmission of SARS-COV-2 infection among humans." **and**
"In conclusion, we propose that curcumin could be used as a supportive therapy in the treatment of COVID-19 disease in any clinical settings to circumvent the lethal effects of SARS-CoV-2." [48]

k. Online Dossier of Scientific Research Findings:

https://theantiviraldiet.com/ingredient-%2326-%2B-research

Ingredient #27 GINGEROL

6-Gingerol, 8-Gingerol & 10-Gingerol

a. Found as:

*Key Ingredient in **Ginger** (Zingiber Officinale)*

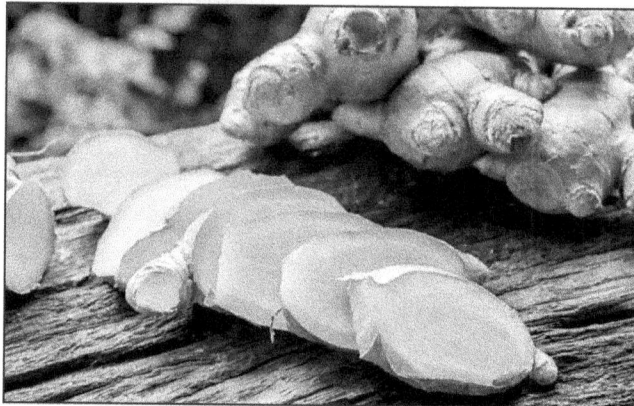

b. Widely Used as:

A Spice Ingredient in Indian, Chinese, Vietnamese, Korean, Vietnamese & other South Asian Cuisine

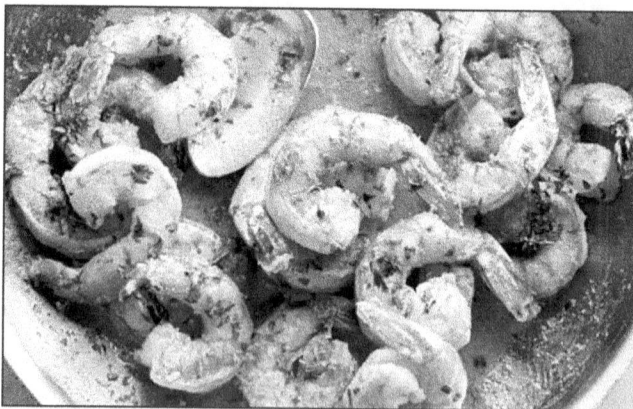

c. Also Popular in:

Medicinal Tea Infusions and as a Natural Flavouring

d. Effect upon Viruses:
Anti-Viral Action evidenced against Human Respiratory Syncytial Virus, Chikungunya Virus, Influenza A Virus, Norwalk Virus, Herpes Simplex Virus, Hepatitis C Virus

e. Impact on Immunity:
Main Impact of Gingerol is Direct Anti-Viral Action qv. d. Has Direct Effect upon Regulatory Immune Mechanisms

f. Additional Information:
Also Anti-Inflammatory, Antioxidant and Bactericidal. It is currently being researched **re:** SARS-CoV-2 Virus

g. Recommended Daily Intake: Not Applicable

h. Human Safety: Non-Toxic but Excess may be harmful

i. Research Quote - Potential against COVID-19:
"*Phytocompound 6-gingerol possesses excellent drug likeliness with zero violations and very good pharmacokinetic properties with the highest binding affinity ranging from -2.8764 KJ/mol to -15.7591 KJ/mol with various COVID-19 viral protein targets. Our study reveals that 6-gingerol from ginger could act as a promising drug of choice to treat COVID-19.*" [49]

"*The chemical constituents from pepper such as Piperdardiine, Piperanine, and from ginger like 8-Gingerol, 10-Gingerol are significantly active against COVID-19 which are useful for further development.*" [50]

j. Research Quote - Anti-Viral against SARS-CoV-2:
"*Eight compounds from Alpinia officinarum and Ginger bind with high in silico affinity to closed PLpro conformer, and hence are potential SARS-CoV-2 PLpro inhibitors.*" [51]

k. Online Dossier of Scientific Research Findings:
https://theantiviraldiet.com/ingredient-%2327-%2B-research

Ingredient #28 PIPERINE

a. <u>Found in</u>:
Black Pepper (Piper Nigrum) & **Long Pepper**
(both Piper Longum L. and Piper Officinarum)

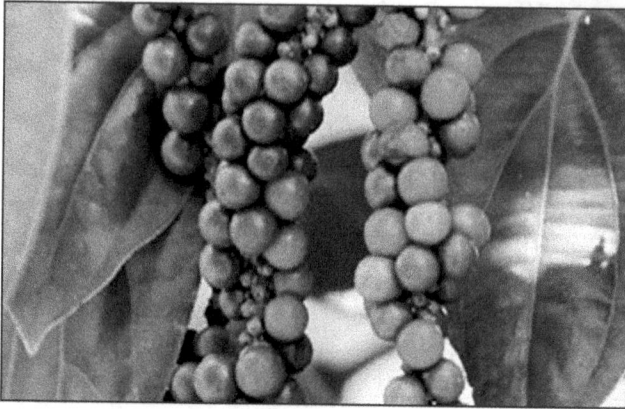

b. <u>Widely Used as</u>:
Pepper is the Most Basic Food Seasoning alongside
Salt - contains nutrients Vitamin K, Iron & Manganese

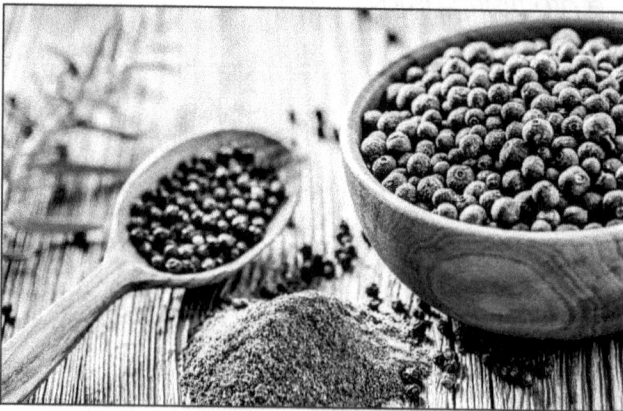

c. <u>Historically</u>:
Used since 2000 BCE and traded with as 'Black Gold'

d. Effect upon Viruses:

Anti-Viral Action evidenced against Dengue Virus, Ebola Virus, Vesicular Stomatitis Virus, Human Parainfluenza Virus, Coxsackievirus Type B3, Influenza A Virus, Human Rhinovirus Type 2 *inter alia*

e. Impact on Immunity:

Main Impact of Piperine is Direct Anti-Viral Action *qv.* **d.**

f. Additional Information:

It is currently being researched **re:** SARS-CoV-2 Virus

g. Recommended Daily Intake: Not Applicable

h. Human Safety: Non-Toxic but Excess can be harmful

i. Research Quote – Anti-Viral against SARS-CoV-2:

"This binding of these molecules will be helpful in inhibiting the replication of the viral proteins with specific hindrances upon their mutarotation. For both the viral targets, Piperine performed well with its highest binding affinity of -7.8 and -7.3 kcal/mol for SARS-CoV-2 Spro and Mpro, respectively. Hence, the study proposes Piperine as an active molecule for the inhibition of SARS-CoV-2. Since this study is performed computationally, therefore, it requires wet-lab experiments in-vivo as well as in-vitro for further validation." [52]

j. Research Quote – SARS-CoV-2 Therapeutic Agent:

*"Our study exhibited that curcumin, nimbin, withaferin A, **piperine**, mangiferin, thebaine, berberine, and andrographolide have significant binding affinity towards spike glycoprotein of SARS-CoV-2 and ACE2 receptor and may be useful as a therapeutic and/or prophylactic agent for restricting viral attachment to the host cells."* [53]

k. Online Dossier of Scientific Research Findings:

https://theantiviraldiet.com/ingredient-%2328-%2B-research

Ingredient #29 ROSEMARY

a. Known as:
Salvia Rosmarinus, a member of the Mint family – Rosmarinic Acid & Oleanolic Acid are Ingredients

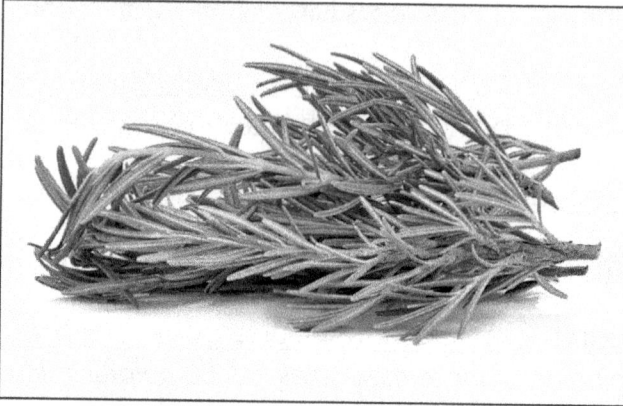

b. Widely Used as:
*A Seasoning for Meats, Pasta Dishes, Stuffings **et al**.*
A Herbal Tea Infusion - also used as an Essential Oil

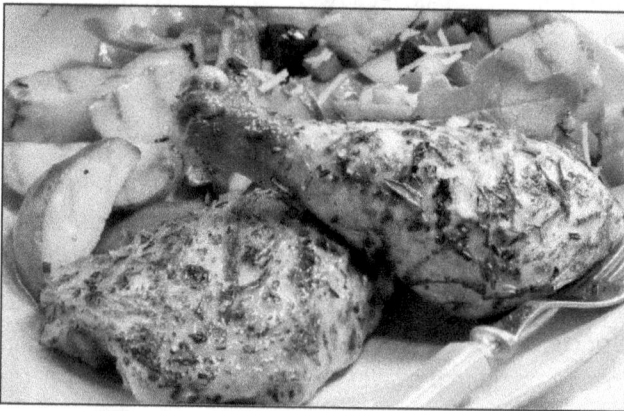

c. Historically:
First mentioned on Cuneiform Tablets circa 5000 BCE

d. Effect upon Viruses:

Anti-Viral Action evidenced against Enterovirus 71, Hepatitis A Virus, Hepatitis B Virus, Hepatitis C Virus, Herpes Simplex Virus Type 1, Herpes Simplex Virus Type 2, Japanese Encephalitis, Human Immunodeficiency Virus, Influenza A Virus *inter alia*

e. Impact on Immunity:

Main Impact of Rosemary is Direct Anti-Viral Action *qv.* d.

f. Additional Information:

Also Anti-Inflammatory, Antioxidant and Bactericidal.

g. Recommended Daily Intake: Not Applicable

h. Human Safety: Non-Toxic but Excess can be harmful

i. Research Quote – Immuno-Modulatory Effect:

"A number of studies have been found a stimulatory effect of rosemary and its active compounds on the immune system in vitro and animal study, but there is a lack of evidence in humans for supporting this. The results demonstrated the potential of rosemary and its main active components as dietary ingredients with immunomodulatory functionality. Human studies should be performed and a double-blind randomized controlled trial would be ideal." [54]

j. Research Quote – Anti-Viral against SARS-CoV-2:

[Regarding tests with Rosmarinic Acid from Rosemary]
"We will expect that if its anti-SARS-CoV-2 activity is validated in human clinical trials, these two drugs may be developed as an effective antiviral therapeutics towards infected patients in this outbreak and pandemic situation of COVID-19." [55]

k. Online Dossier of Scientific Research Findings:

https://theantiviraldiet.com/ingredient-%2329-%2B-research

Ingredient #30 OREGANO & SAGE

a. Known as:

Origanum Vulgare and *Salvia Officinalis* - both
from the Mint family, like Rosemary (**Ingr.#29**)

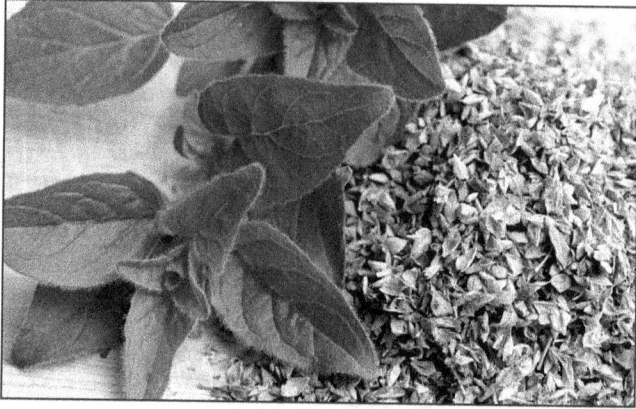

b. Essential Herbs:

Oregano is perhaps most famous as "the Pizza Herb"
Sage is in 'Sage & Onion Stuffing' in Chicken/Turkey

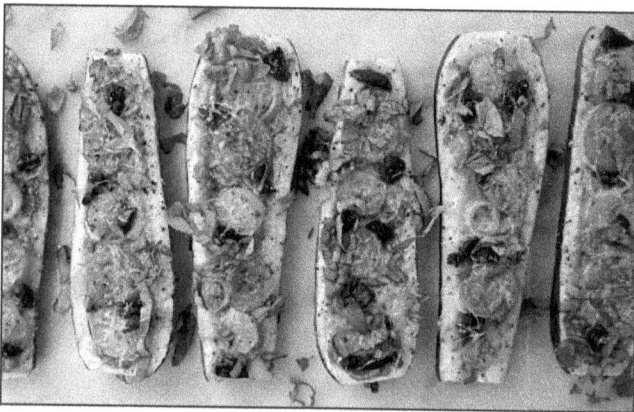

c. Also Found as:

Essential Oils - Dioscorides mentions in 1st Century CE

d. Effect upon Viruses:
Anti-Viral Action evidenced against Human Immunodeficiency Virus, Herpes Simplex Virus Type 1, Vesicular Stomatitis Virus, Norovirus, SARS-CoV-1 [Oregano] *inter alia*

e. Impact on Immunity:
Main Impact of of Oregano and Sage is Direct Anti-Viral Action *qv.* **d.** Oregano is linked with Respiratory Health

f. Additional Information:
Both also Anti-Inflammatory, Antioxidant and Bactericidal. They are currently being researched **re:** SARS-CoV-2 Virus

g. Recommended Daily Intake: Not Applicable

h. Human Safety: Non-Toxic but Excess can be harmful

i. Research Quote - Immuno-Modulatory Effect:
"Supercritical extracts from edible herbs like oregano and sage presented important antiviral activities against herpes simplex type 1, overall extracts obtained in separator 1. These extracts mainly inhibit HSV-1 intracellular replication, although they were also able to disrupt the virus attachment step. Carvacrol and thymol could be pointed out as the compounds responsible for the antiviral activity found in oregano." [56]

j. Research Quote - Effect upon SARS-CoV-2:
"Study of the antiviral effects of plant extracts is aimed at developing new strategies in the treatment of different viral infections. [...] From our results with sage it is clear that cultivated sage, especially fraction 144/5, deserves further investigation to evaluate its antiviral potential and active principals against different viruses." [57]

k. Online Dossier of Scientific Research Findings:
https://theantiviraldiet.com/ingredient-%2330-%2B-research

Ingredient #31 PEPPERMINT

a. Known as:

*Mentha Piperita and also as **Mentha Balsamea** - like Ingrs.#29 and #30, it is from the Mint Family*

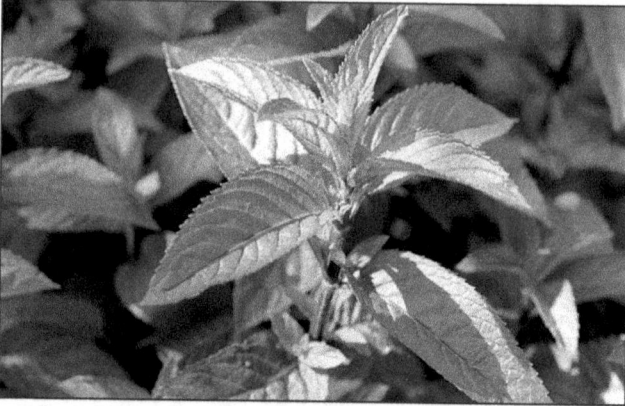

b. Widely Used as:

Herbal Tea Infusion, especially good for Digestion & Popular Confectionery Flavouring; Sweets & Chocolate

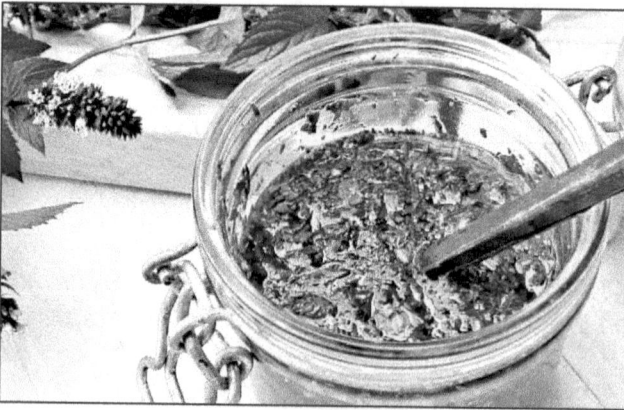

c. World Fact:

Over 90% of all Peppermint comes out of Morocco

d. Effect upon Viruses:
Anti-Viral Action evidenced against Human Immuno-deficiency Virus, Herpes Simplex Virus Type 1, Herpes Simplex Virus Type 2, Newcastle Disease Virus, Vaccinia Virus, West Nile Virus, Semliki Forest Virus *inter alia*

e. Impact on Immunity:
Main Impact of Peppermint is Direct Anti-Viral Action *qv.* **d.**

f. Additional Information:
Also Anti-Inflammatory, Antioxidant and Bactericidal. It is currently being researched **re**: SARS-CoV-2 Virus

g. Recommended Daily Intake: Not Applicable

h. Human Safety: Non-Toxic but Excess can be harmful

i. Research Quote - Essential Oils as Anti-Virals:
" The essential oils (EOs) and their chemical constituents are known to be active against a wide range of viruses. Oxygenated monoterpenes and sesquiterpenes present in EOs contribute to their antiviral effect. Since the new strain of coronavirus, now named SARS-CoV-2 (Severe Acute Respiratory Syndrome Coronavirus), is still not completely understood, it is not yet possible to find which EOs will offer the best level of protection." [58]

j. Research Quote - Anti-Viral against HIV-1:
"Aqueous extracts from Lamiaceae can drastically and rapidly reduce the infectivity of HIV-1 virions at non-cytotoxic concentrations. An extract-induced enhancement of the virion's density prior to its surface engagement appears to be the most likely mode of action. By harbouring also a strong activity against herpes simplex virus type 2, these extracts may provide a basis for the development of novel virucidal topical microbicides." [59]

k. Online Dossier of Scientific Research Findings:
https://theantiviraldiet.com/ingredient-%2331-%2B-research

Ingredient #32 BASIL & HOLY BASIL

a. Known as:

Ocimum Basilicum and *Ocimum Sanctum* (Tulsi) – two more herbs in **AVD** from the Mint Family (Lamiaceae)

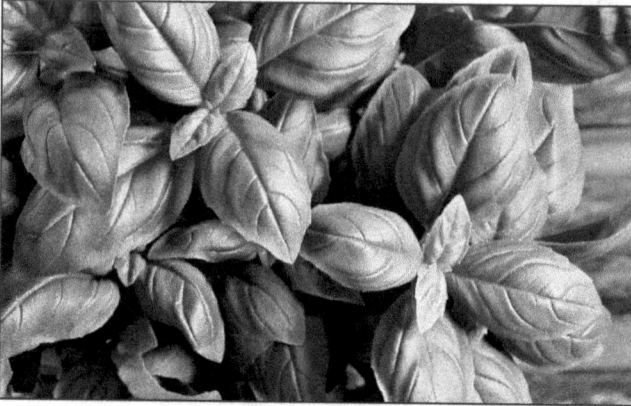

b. Main Uses:

*While Basil is a Key Herb in Italian Cuisine (Pesto **et al.**) Holy Basil has Religious (Hindu) and Medicinal Uses*

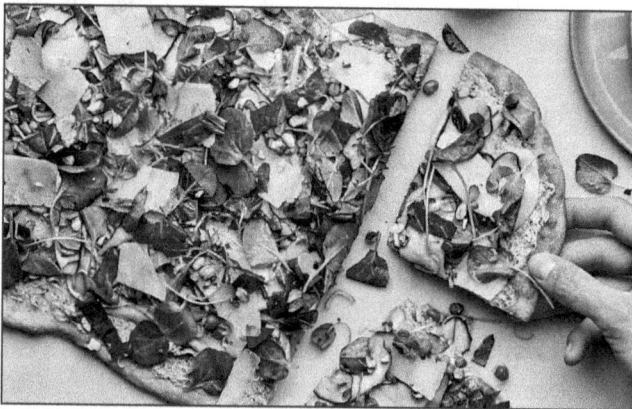

c. Etymology:

'Basil comes' from Greek 'Basilikón Phutón' (Kingly Plant)

d. Effect upon Viruses:
Anti-Viral Action evidenced against Hepatitis B Virus, Herpes Simplex Virus Type 1, Coxsackievirus B1, Adenoviruses, Enterovirus-71 & Influenza H9N2 Virus

e. Impact on Immunity:
Main Impact of Basil/Tulsi is Direct Anti-Viral Action *qv.* **d.** - Tulsi increases Natural Killer Cells and T Helper Cells

f. Additional Information:
Both also Anti-Inflammatory, Antioxidant and Bactericidal. They are currently being researched **re:** SARS-CoV-2 Virus

g. Recommended Daily Intake: Not Applicable

h. Human Safety: Non-Toxic but Excess can be harmful

i. Research Quote - Broad-Based Anti-Viral Action:
"In the present study, extracts and purified components of OB [Ocimum Basilicum] *were used to identify possible antiviral activities against DNA viruses (herpes viruses (HSV), adenoviruses (ADV) and hepatitis B virus) and RNA viruses (coxsackievirus B1 (CVB1) and enterovirus 71 (EV71)). 2. The results show that crude aqueous and ethanolic extracts of OB and selected purified components, namely apigenin, linalool and ursolic acid, exhibit a broad spectrum of antiviral activity."* [60]

j. Research Quote - Anti-Viral against H9N2 Virus:
"The crude extract and terpenoid isolated from the leaves of O. sanctum [Tulsi] *and polyphenol from A. arabica has shown promising antiviral properties against H9N2 virus. Future investigations are necessary to formulate combinations of these compounds for the broader antiviral activity against H9N2 viruses and evaluate them in chickens."* [61]

k. Online Dossier of Scientific Research Findings:
https://theantiviraldiet.com/ingredient-%2332-%2B-research

PLANTS & FLOWERS

THE ONLY DIFFERENCE between these ingredients and those included in the preceding section of the diet, is that the ones presented here are almost exclusively suitable as the constituents of beverages and not as ingredients for actual meals. Some of them are also commonly available in root or stalk form, like Galangal and Ginger in the preceding sub-section, but they are *most suitable* to be used within medicinal drinks. In fact, every single one of the ingredients in this section can be made into a hot drink, either by infusing (adding the ingredient to boiled water) or by boiling/simmering in water for a period of time). The only difference is that in the former case, flowers or leaves are generally utilized, while in the latter, roots or bark are usually suitable. What may be apparent, to at least some readers, is that half of the dietary elements presented here are often used in Traditional Chinese Medicine (TCM) - thus have a long history of practical, remedial use.

Glycyrrhizin - identifying the exact compound in this instance - is the most active ingredient in Liquorice, which is still available as sticks at some confectioners. It eases heartburn and other digestive problems, is an anti-inflammatory and is able to resolve respiratory problems, *e.g.* bronchial infection.

Ginseng is described as an 'Adaptogenic' compound, meaning that is able to stabilize physiological processes and encourage homeostasis (a stable internal state) of the body. It has been evidenced to be an antioxidant, anti-inflammatory, positively affects memory and has anti-cancer effects.

Astragalus is perhaps one of the most famed immune-stimulating natural ingredients, apart from Echinacea (*qv.*) and it was first identified (as a genus) by Carl Linnaeus in 1753. It contains saponins and isoflavone flavonoids, which are traditionally used to increase lactation for nursing mothers. It is an antioxidant, and is used to alleviate stress and insomnia *et al.*

Andrographis has been a widely used medicinal plant, used for many conditions – including cancer, diabetes, leprosy, bronchitis, influenza, dysentery and malaria. Compounds of the plant have been reported as being anti-microbial, anti-inflammatory, anti-oxidant, anti-diabetic and anti-infective.

Cat's Claw – also known as *Uncaria Tomentosa* – has been a traditional medicine in South American countries for as long as two thousand years. Evidence has emerged of its ability to ease the symptoms of osteoarthritis and rheumatoid arthritis. It has long been known to be an immunostimulant.

Dandelion and *Burdock* are both used in TCM, though for different purposes. Both of these plants contain sesquiterpene lactones, which research has shown to have a number of qualities, including being bactericidal and fungicidal. Burdock leaves also contain Caffeic Acid and Chlorogenic Acid.

Lemon Balm is a lemon-scented herb that is from the same family as mint, popular as a tea infusion. It has had many traditional uses but has only more recently been discovered to have anti-oxidative, anti-bacterial and anti-viral qualities.

Echinacea is a flower – also known as the Coneflower – native to North America. It is known that it was used by some American Indians for cold symptoms (cough, sore throat) and for pain relief. It is now well-known for its immunostimulatory qualities and for being anti-oxidative and anti-inflammatory.

St. John's Wort, also named as *Hypericum Perforatum*, has become quite widely known as a natural anti-depressant. However, an extract called 'St. John's Oil' has been used in the treatment of wounds for centuries. It has potent anti-bacterial, anti-oxidant and (discovered most recently) anti-viral qualities.

Hibiscus is a large genus of plants containing a couple of hundred species. *Hibiscus Sabdariffa* and *Hibiscus Rosa-Sinensis* are appreciated as tea infusions, due to their positive effects upon human health. Both these Hibiscus varieties are anti-oxidative, anti-bacterial and have anti-viral effects.

Other ingredients, like Pau D'Arco, were considered but insufficient evidence exists for inclusion at the present time.

127

Ingredient #33 GLYCYRRHIZIN

a. Found as:

*Most Potent Ingredient in **Liquorice** (or **Licorice**)*
Also known as Glycyrrhizic/Glycyrrhizinic Acid

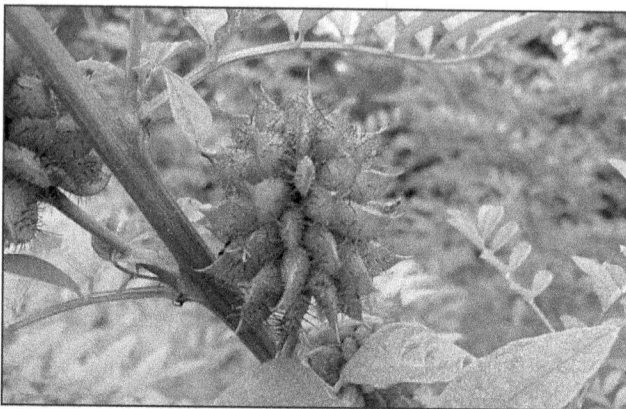

b. Widely Available as:

Liquorice Sticks, Liquorice Powder, Liquorice Tea
- although Liquorice Candy is Most Popular Form

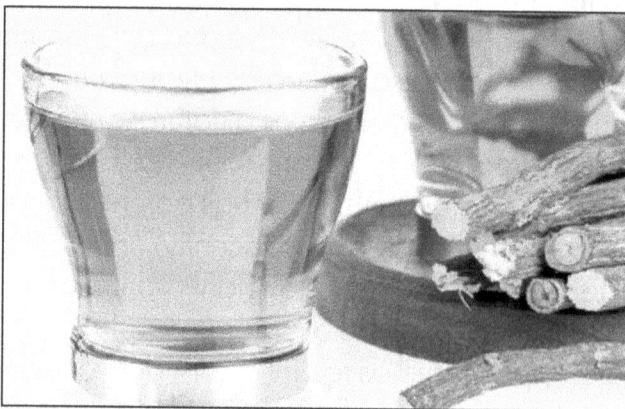

c. Worth Knowing:

*Liquorice also contains **Anethole** (3%) [qv. Ingr.#52]*

d. Effect upon Viruses:

Anti-Viral Action evidenced against SARS-CoV-1, Hepatitis B Virus, Hepatitis C Virus, Encephalitis, Herpes Simplex Virus, Influenza A Virus, Human Immunodeficiency Virus (HIV-1 & HIV-2), Respiratory Syncytial Virus, Arboviruses, Vaccinia Virus, Vesicular Stomatitis Virus, Varicella Zoster Virus & Kaposi's Sarcoma-Associated Herpesvirus

e. Impact on Immunity:

Main Impact of Glycyrrhizin is Direct Anti-Viral Action qv. d.

f. Additional Information:

It enhances Immune Response and regulates Inflammation

g. Recommended Daily Intake: Not Applicable

h. Human Safety: Non-Toxic but Excess can be harmful

i. Research Quote – Immuno-Modulatory Effects:

"Glycyrrhizin has cytokine-modulating activity, it is not an immunosuppressant like glucocorticoids, and may even enhance the immune response. Therefore, glycyrrhizin is expected to be used in the early stages of disease and can be administered for a longer time, with fewer side effects; this approach holds promise for preventing or attenuating excessive cytokine storms in patients with COVID-19." [62]

j. Research Quote – Potential against COVID-19:

"The membrane and cytoplasmic effects of GLR [glycyrrhizic acid], coupled with its long-established medical use as a relatively safe drug, make GLR a good candidate to be tested against the SARS-CoV-2 coronavirus, alone and in combination with other drugs. [...] Based on this analysis, we conclude that GLR should be further considered and rapidly evaluated for the treatment of patients with COVID-19." [63]

k. Online Dossier of Scientific Research Findings:

https://theantiviraldiet.com/ingredient-%2333-%2B-research

Ingredient #34 GINSENG

a. Known as:

Panax Ginseng (Korean Ginseng) - Other Forms include **Panax Notoginseng** *and* **Panax Quinquefolius**

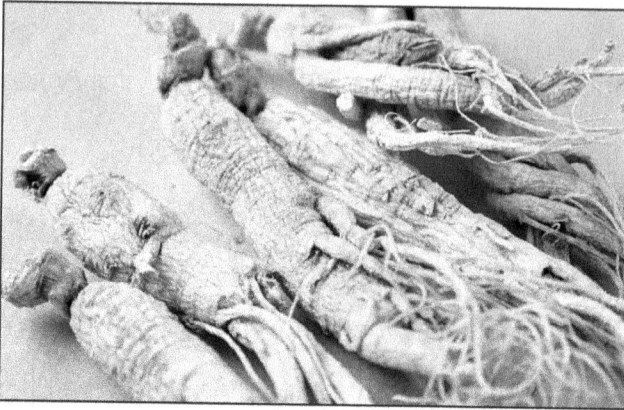

b. Used in:

Soups and other Dishes in Korea, as the Central Ingredient of Ginseng Tea - also as a Medicine

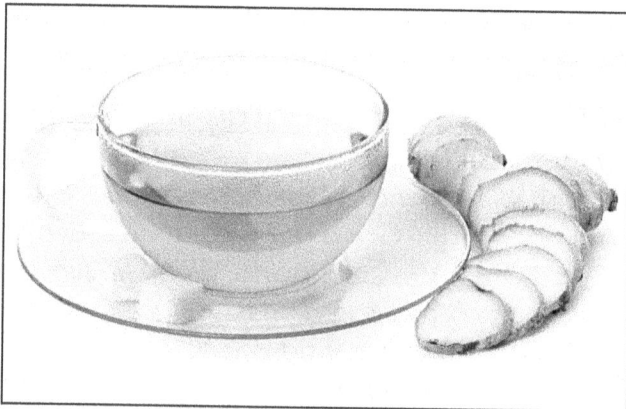

c. Etymology:

'Panax' means "All-Healing" like the word 'Panacea'

d. Effect upon Viruses:
Anti-Viral Action evidenced against Human Immunodeficiency Virus Type 1, Respiratory Syncytial Virus, Chronic Hepatitis B Virus, Human Norovirus, Rhinovirus, Influenza, Rotaviruses, Enteroviruses, Coxsackievirus & SARS-CoV-1

e. Effect on Immune System:
Main Impact of Ginsengs is Direct Anti-Viral Action *qv.* d. although it is known to be an Immunomodulatory Agent

f. Additional Information:
Also Anti-Inflammatory, Antioxidant and Bactericidal. It is currently being researched **re:** SARS-CoV-2 Virus

g. Recommended Daily Intake: Not Applicable

h. Human Safety: Non-Toxic but Excess can be harmful

i. Research Quote – Potential against COVID-19:
" *Ginseng stem-leaf saponins could highly enhance the specific antibody responses for Newcastle disease virus and infectious bronchitis virus. Therefore, Chinese Medicine could also be considered as a choice to enhance host immunity against the infection of COVID-19.* " [2]

j. Research Quote – Anti-Bacterial and Anti-Viral:
" *Ginseng has the functions to strongly tonify the Qi, nourishing lungs and spleen, promoting the secretion of saliva and quenching thirst, strengthening the heart, and calming the mind. Several studies recently report that ginseng can directly kill bacteria and regulate bacterial adhesion, inflammation, cytotoxicity, and hemagglutination. Wang et al. report that ginseng extracts can inhibit different strains of influenza viruses.* " [64]

k. Online Dossier of Scientific Research Findings:
https://theantiviraldiet.com/ingredient-%2334-%2B-research

Ingredient #35 ASTRAGALUS

a. Types used:

Astragalus Membranaceus and *Astragalus Mongholicus*
- out of the Astragalus Genus, with over 3000 species

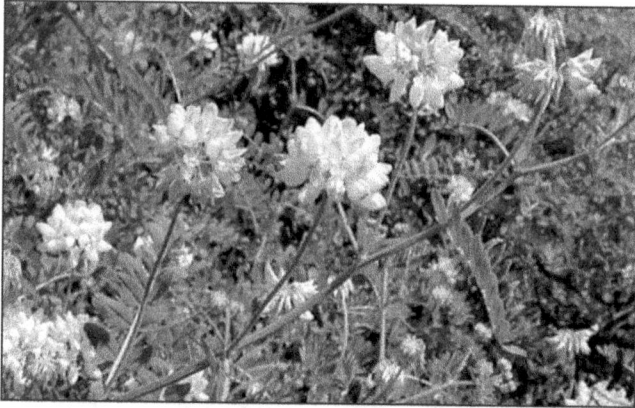

b. Used as:

*'Huang Qi' (Milkvetch) is a Medicinal Herb used
for many centuries in Traditional Chinese Medicine*

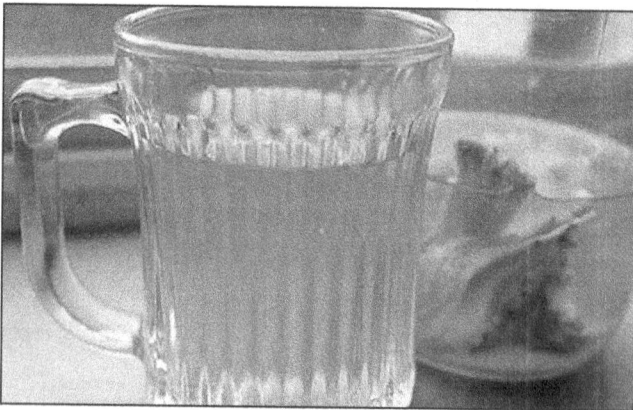

c. World View:

In China it is even given as Injection or Intravenously

d. Effect upon Viruses:
Anti-Viral Action evidenced against Influenza Virus, Herpes Simplex Viruses. Key Effect is on Immune System *qv.* **e.**

e. Impact on Immunity:
Increases Immunological Functions; like Maitake, Reishi & Shiitake, it contains some Bioactive Polysaccharides

f. Additional Information:
Also Anti-Inflammatory, Antioxidant and Bactericidal. It is currently being researched re: SARS-CoV-2 Virus

g. Recommended Daily Intake: Not Applicable

h. Human Safety: Non-Toxic but Excess can be harmful

i. Research Quote - Anti-Viral against H9 Virus:
"Antiviral activity of Astragalus membranaceus aqueous and methanol root extracts was determined against Avian influenza H9 virus. [...] It was concluded that aqueous and methanol roots extracts of A. membranaceus have antiviral activity and concentrations which were safe may be used for treatment of Avian influenza H9 virus infections." [65]

j. Research Quote - Immuno-Modulatory Effects:
"Similarly, astragalus polysaccharide (APS, 33), the most immuno-reactive substance extracted from Astragalus, are commonly used in immune related diseases. Lately, the antiviral effect of APS was detected in astrocytes infected by HSV-1. Research uncovered that APS could not inhibit the virus directly, but instead it protected astrocytes by promoting immunological function, such as markedly increasing the expression of tumor necrosis factor-a (TNF-a), interleukin6 (IL-6), Toll-like receptor (TLR3), and nuclear factor-κB (NF-κB) provoked by HSV-1." [66]

k. Online Dossier of Scientific Research Findings:
https://theantiviraldiet.com/ingredient-%2335-%2B-research

Ingredient #36 ANDROGRAPHOLIDE

a. Found in:

The Plant **Andrographis Paniculata**, which comes from the Andrographis (False Waterwillows) Genus

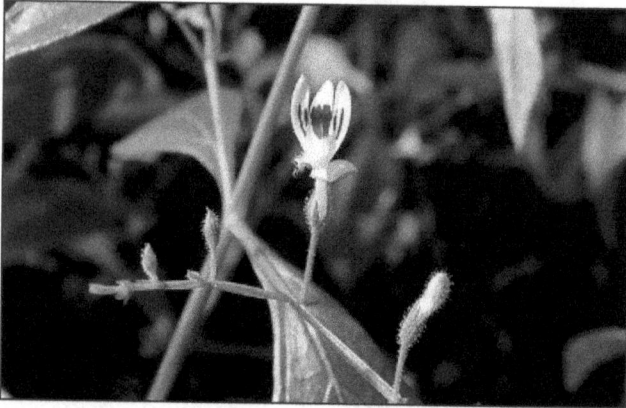

b. Used in:

Traditional Chinese Medicine for a Variety of Conditions including Cancer, Bronchitis, Influenza & Malaria

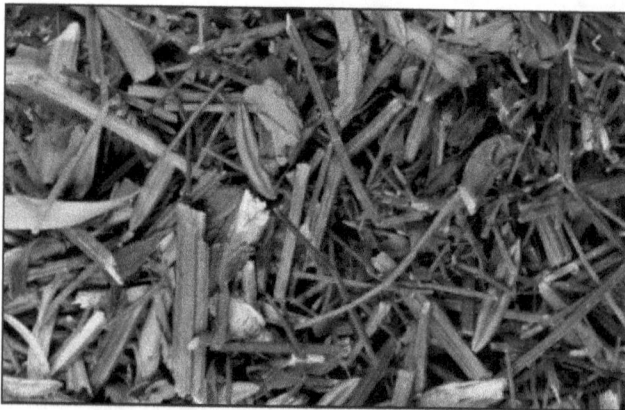

c. Origins:

Native to India, Bengali 'Kalmegh' means "King of Bitters"

d. Effect Upon Viruses:
Anti-Viral Action evidenced against Dengue Virus, Ebola Virus, SARS-CoV-1, Herpes Simple Virus Type 1, Influenza A Virus, Chikungunya Virus, Hepatitis B Virus, Hepatitis C Virus, Epstein-Barr Virus, Human Papillomavirus, Human Immunodeficiency Virus (HIV-1) *inter alia*

e. Impact on Immunity:
Improves Innate & Adaptive Immune Response; Increases Lymphocyte Creation, enhances Natural Killer Cell Activity

f. Additional Information:
It is currently being researched **re:** SARS-CoV-2 Virus

g. Recommended Daily Intake: Not Applicable

h. Human Safety: Non-Toxic but Excess can be harmful

i. Research Quote - Potential against COVID-19:
"The study suggests the strong interaction of the andrographolide and its derivative 14-deoxy-11,12-didehydroandrographolide against target proteins associated with COVID-19. Further, network pharmacology analysis elucidated the different pathways of immunomodulation. However, clinical research should be conducted to confirm the current findings." [67]

j. Research Quote - Anti-Viral against SARS-CoV-2:
"This paper evaluates the compound Andrographolide from Andrographis paniculata as a potential inhibitor of the main protease of SARS-COV-2 (Mpro) through in silico studies such as molecular docking, target analysis, toxicity prediction and ADME prediction. Andrographolide was docked successfully in the binding site of SARS-CoV-2 Mpro. Computational approaches also predicts this molecule to have good solubility, pharmacodynamics property and target accuracy." [68]

k. Online Dossier of Scientific Research Findings:
https://theantiviraldiet.com/ingredient-%2336-%2B-research

Ingredient #37 CAT'S CLAW

a. Known as:

Uña de Gato or *Unha de Gato* (Spanish/Portuguese)
- most importantly refers to Plant **Uncaria Tomentosa**

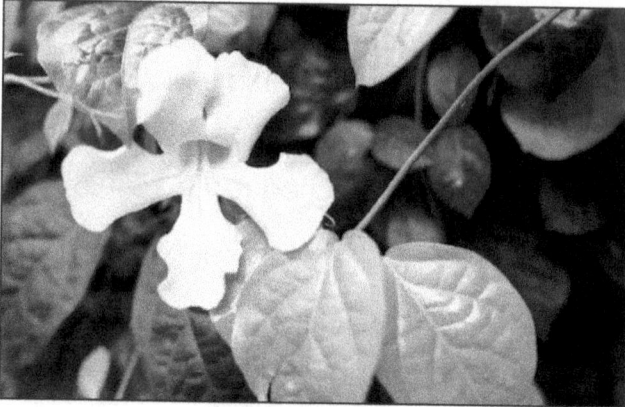

b. Traditionally:

Grown in Amazon Rain Forest - used for a Variety of Conditions including Infections, Cancer, Arthritis **et al.**

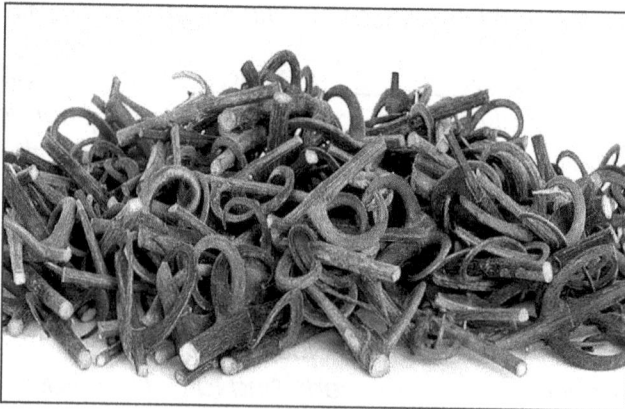

c. Etymology:

So-called because of its Cat-like Claws at Base of Leaves

d. Effect upon Viruses:
Anti-Viral Action evidenced against Dengue Fever Virus Type 2, Herpes Simplex Virus Type 1, Herpes Simplex Virus Type 2, Epstein-Barr Virus & Hepatitis Viruses

e. Impact on Immunity:
Improves Immune Response; via Increased Proliferation of Lymphocytes and via management of Inflammatory factors

f. Additional Information:
Also Anti-Inflammatory, Antioxidant and Bactericidal. It is currently being researched **re:** SARS-CoV-2 Virus. It has a long History of use as a Traditional Medicine.

g. Recommended Daily Intake: Not Applicable

h. Human Safety: Non-Toxic but Excess can be harmful

i. Research Quote - Potential against COVID-19:
"The structural bioinformatics approaches led to the identification of three bioactive compounds of Uncaria tomentosa (Speciophylline, Cadambine and Proanthocyanidin B2) with potential therapeutic effects by strong interaction with 3CLpro. Additionally, in silico drug-likeness indices for these components were calculated and show good predicted therapeutic profiles of these phytochemicals. Our findings suggest the potential effectiveness of Cat's claw as complementary and/or alternative medicine for COVID-19 treatment." [69]

j. Research Quote - Anti-Viral/Immuno-Modulatory:
"The antiviral and immunomodulating in vitro effects from U. tomentosa pentacyclic oxindole alkaloids displayed novel properties regarding therapeutic procedures in Dengue Fever and might be further investigated as a promising candidate for clinical application." [70]

k. Online Dossier of Scientific Research Findings:
https://theantiviraldiet.com/ingredient-%2337-%2B-research

Ingredient #38 DANDELION & BURDOCK

a. Known as:

Taraxacum Officinale and **Arctium** - *have several traits in common, both from the Asteraceae Family*

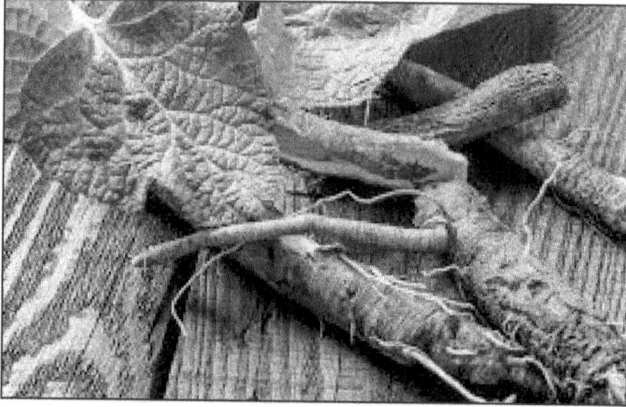

b. Multiple Uses:

Dandelion Leaves are used in Salad, Burdock Root also as Food. All parts of both plants for Medicinal Purposes

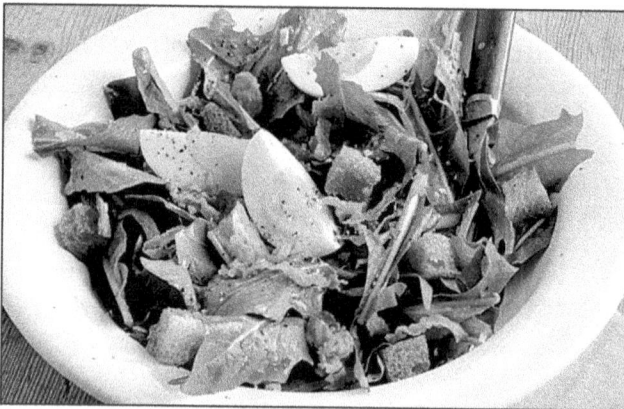

c. Traditionally:

'Dandelion & Burdock' is a popular Sparkling Cordial

d. Effect upon Viruses:
Anti-Viral Action evidenced against Influenza Viruses, Hepatitis B Virus, Dengue Fever Virus Type 2, Herpes Simplex Virus Type 1 & Herpes Simplex Virus Type 2

e. Impact on Immunity:
Main Impact of these both is Direct Anti-Viral Action *qv.* **d.**

f. Additional Information:
Both also Anti-Inflammatory, Antioxidant and Bactericidal. They are currently being researched **re**: SARS-CoV-2 Virus

g. Recommended Daily Intake: Not Applicable

h. Human Safety: Non-Toxic but Excess can be harmful

i. Research Quote - Anti-Viral Effect of Dandelion:
"The antiviral activity of dandelion extracts indicates that a component or components of these extracts possess anti-influenza virus properties. Mechanisms of reduction of viral growth in MDCK or A549 cells by dandelion involve inhibition on virus replication." [71]

j. Research Quote - Burdock as Immuno-Modulatory:
"The roots and leaves of Arctium lappa (burdock) have been used for different therapeutic purposes, especially for diseases linked to chronic inflammation. [...] The present study was designed to evaluate and compare the immunomodulatory activities of root extract of burdock and leaves extract of burdock in vitro. [...] Although both root and leaves extract of burdock had similar immunomodulatory effects in vitro, stronger immunomodulatory effects seen in root extract of burdock."
and
"[W]e suggest that root of burdock is better option than leaves of burdock in modulation immune responses and inflammations." [72]

k. Online Dossier of Scientific Research Findings:
https://theantiviraldiet.com/ingredient-%2338-%2B-research

Ingredient #39 LEMON BALM

a. Known as:

Melissa Officinalis - like *Peppermint, Sage, Rosemary & Oregano* - is also part of the Mint Family (Lamiaceae)

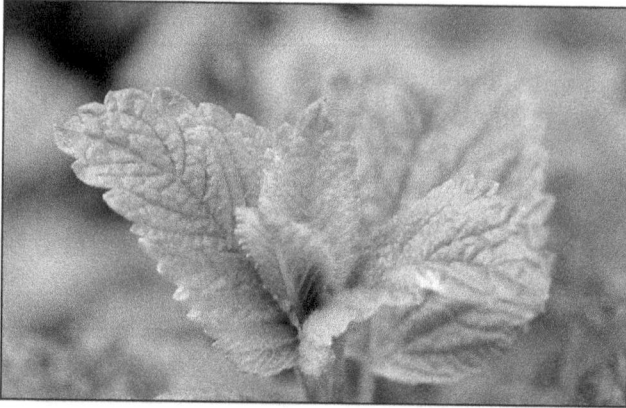

b. Used as:

The Main Ingredient in a Tea Infusion, although also as a Herb with Fish and in Pesto. An Essential Oil too

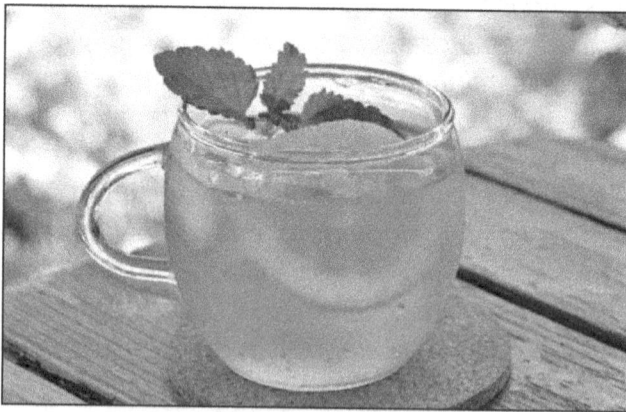

c. Historically:

Lemon Balm has been cultivated since the 16th Century

d. Effect upon Viruses:

Anti-Viral Action evidenced against Newcastle Virus, Vaccinia Virus, Semliki Forest Virus, Herpes Simplex Virus Type 2, Human Immunodeficiency Virus (HIV-1) *inter alia*

e. Impact on Immunity:

Main Impact of Lemon Balm is Direct Anti-Viral Action *qv.* d.

f. Additional Information:

Also Anti-Inflammatory, Antioxidant and Bactericidal. It is currently being researched **re:** SARS-CoV-2 Virus

g. Recommended Daily Intake: Not Applicable

h. Human Safety: Non-Toxic but Excess can be harmful

i. Research Quote - Anti-Viral against Influenza:

"*Lemon balm derivatives are going to acquire a novelty as natural and potent remedy for treatment of viral infections since the influenza viruses are developing resistance to the current antivirals widely. [...] In conclusion, the findings of the study showed that lemon balm essential oil could inhibit influenza virus replication through different replication cycle steps especially throughout the direct interaction with the virus particles.*" [73]

j. Research Quote - Immuno-Modulatory Effects:

"*The effect of an extract from Melissa officinalis on immune response in mice was analysed using the cytotoxicity test in three dilutions (undiluted extract and extract diluted 10 and 100 times) [...] The immunostimulating activity of the extract was compared with that of a synthetic compound - levamisole, which influence on the immune system is well known. The present results confirm the effect of water extracts from leaves of Melissa on the immune system, in both humoral and cellular response.*" [74]

k. Online Dossier of Scientific Research Findings:

https://theantiviraldiet.com/ingredient-%2339-%2B-research

Ingredient #40 ECHINACEA

a. Known as:

Echinacea Purpurea - *also called a 'Coneflower' - is from the Echinacea genus in the Daisy Family*

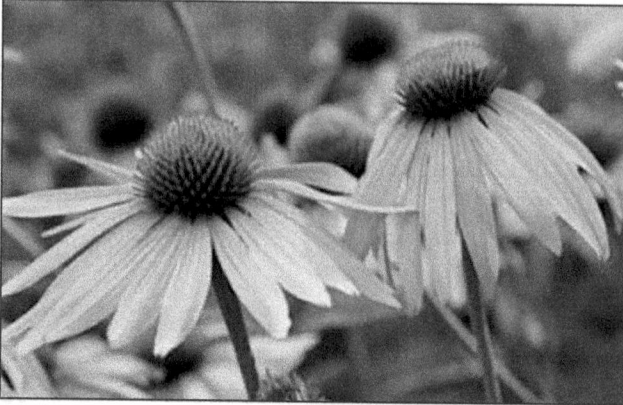

b. Used as:

Herbal Tea Infusion, Tinctures ; Active Ingredients are more active in the Fruit & Flowers than Leaves & Roots

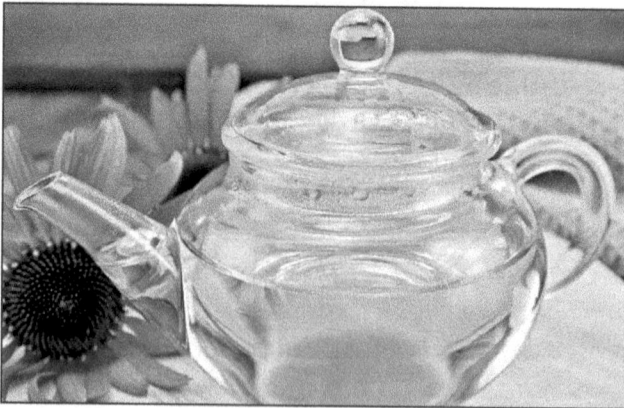

c. Cultivation:

It is only grown in Central and Eastern North America

d. Effect upon Viruses:

Anti-Viral Action evidenced against SARS-CoV-1, MERS-Cov, Influenza A Virus, Influenza B Virus, Respiratory Syncytial Virus, Rhinoviruses, Herpes Simplex Virus Type 1, Herpes Simplex Virus Type 2 *inter alia*

e. Impact on Immunity:

Stimulates Macrophages and other Cells in the Innate Immune System; increases Lymphocytes & CD4 Cells

f. Additional Information:

Also Anti-Inflammatory, Antioxidant and Bactericidal. It is currently being researched **re**: SARS-CoV-2 Virus

g. Recommended Daily Intake: Not Applicable

h. Human Safety: Non-Toxic but Excess can be harmful

i. Research Quote - Anti-Viral against MERS/SARS:

"Finally, antiviral activity was not restricted to common cold coronaviruses, as the highly pathogenic SARS- and MERS-CoVs were inactivated at comparable concentrations. Conclusions: These results suggest that Echinacea purpurea preparations, such as Echinaforce, could be effective as prophylactic treatment for all CoVs, including newly occurring strains, such as SARS-CoV-2." [75]

j. Research Quote - Potential against COVID-19:

"The present study is one such work aimed to test Echinacea purpurea as a possible inhibitor, currently in the market to control and decrease the infection [COVID-19] as quickly as possible. Thus, with reference to the above results, Echinacea purpurea can be used against the COVID-19 (nCoV-2019). In addition, to that key technologies can help to address the nCoV-2019." [76]

k. Online Dossier of Scientific Research Findings:

https://theantiviraldiet.com/ingredient-%2340-%2B-research

Ingredient #41 ST. JOHN'S WORT

a. Known as:

Hypericum Perforatum, from the Family Hypericaceae - its Key Active Ingredients are Hyperforin & Hypericin

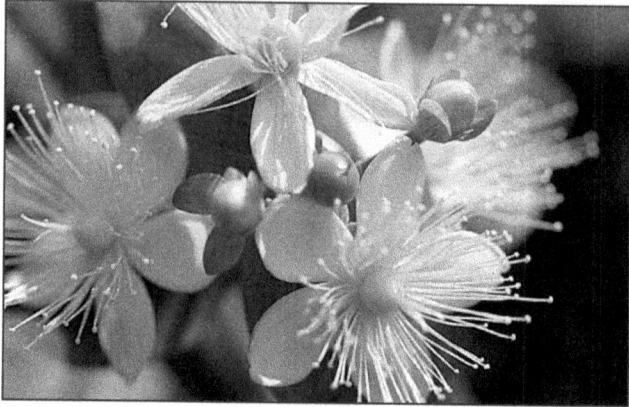

b. Used as:

A Traditional Medicine, dating back to the Romans - popular for Tea Infusions and also as 'St. John's Oil'

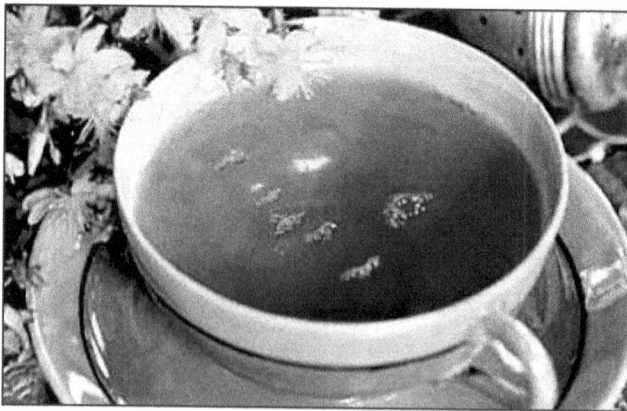

c. Also Used as:

Anti-depressant - shown to have Measurable Effects

d. Effect upon Viruses:
Anti-Viral Action evidenced against Chronic Hepatitis C Virus, Infectious Bronchitis Virus (Prototype Coronavirus), Human Immunodeficiency Virus (HIV-1) *inter alia*

e. Impact on Immunity:
Main Impact of St. John's W. is Direct Anti-Viral Action *qv.* d.

f. Additional Information:
Also Anti-Inflammatory, Antioxidant and Bactericidal. It is currently being researched **re**: SARS-CoV-2 Virus

g. Recommended Daily Intake: Not Applicable

h. Human Safety: Non-Toxic but Excess can be harmful

i. Research Quote - Calming the 'Cytokine Storm':
"*In conclusion, we firmly believe that the anti-inflammatory SJW/HPF [St. John's Wort/Hypericum Perforatum] treatment deserves evaluation in COVID-19 patients. Such a treatment, that offers the additional advantages of being orally administrable, well tolerated, and inexpensive, holds considerable promise to prevent or limit the effects of the cytokine storm through the simultaneous inhibition of NF-κB, JAK/STAT, and MAPK pathways, that is, the three majors signaling and transduction pathways involved in cytokine-induced local and systemic inflammatory changes.*" [77]

j. Research Quote - Potential against COVID-19:
"*This study provides a lead to the possibility of natural anthraquinones being used as treatment for COVID-19, but as this study has been carried out using blind molecular docking method, detailed in vivo and in vitro experiments are required to be carried out to gauge the applicability and toxicity of these anthraquinones.*" [78]

k. Online Dossier of Scientific Research Findings:
https://theantiviraldiet.com/ingredient-%2341-%2B-research

Ingredient #42 HIBISCUS

a. Known as:

Hibiscus Rosa-sinensis - Flowering Plant out of several hundred species in the Malvaceae (Mallow) Family

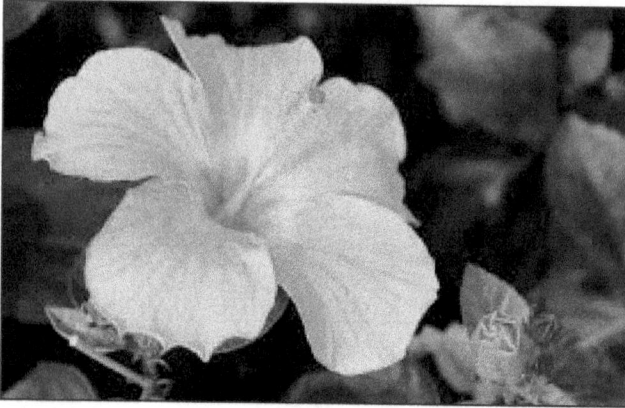

b. Used as:

Popular Tea Infusion, with similar taste to Cranberries - Hibiscus is used in Traditional Ayurvedic Medicine

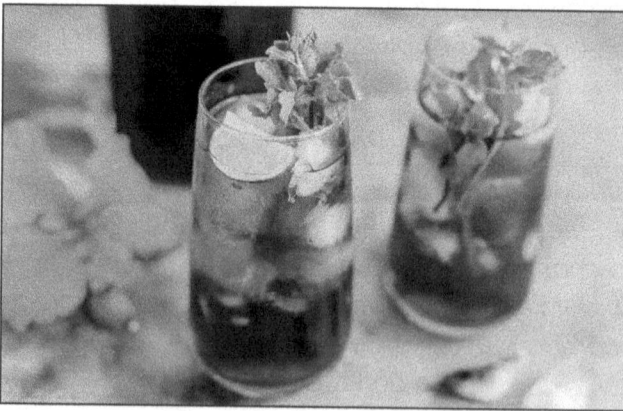

c. Relevant Fact:

Hibiscus sabdariffa also has immuno-enhancing qualities

d. Effect upon Viruses:

Anti-Viral Action evidenced against Human Influenza A Virus, Human Influenza H1N1, Human Influenza H3N2, Measles Virus & Herpes Simplex Viruses Types 1 & 2

e. Impact on Immunity:

Main Impact of Hibiscus is Direct Anti-Viral Action *qv.* d. - It also appears to stimulate Lymphocyte Proliferation

f. Additional Information:

Also Anti-Inflammatory, Antioxidant and Bactericidal. It is currently being researched **re:** SARS-CoV-2 Virus

g. Recommended Daily Intake: Not Applicable

h. Human Safety: Non-Toxic but Excess can be harmful

i. Research Quote - Immuno-Modulatory Effect:

"*The crude extract of H. rosa-sinensis has immunomodulatory activity. [...] HPTLC chromatogram revealed that Hibiscus rosa-sinensis posses alkaloid (Rf 0.93) and flavonoids (Rf 0.02, 0.06, 0.14) on the basis of Rf values. Results of investigation supports for the immunomodulatory activity of H. rosa-sinensis aqueous extract.*" [79]

j. Research Quote - Anti-Viral against Influenza:

"*Here, we analyzed the antiviral activity of hibiscus (Hibiscus sabdariffa L.) tea extract against human IAV and evaluated its potential as a novel anti-IAV drug and a safe inactivating agent for whole inactivated vaccine. The in vitro study revealed that the pH of hibiscus tea extract is acidic, and its rapid and potent antiviral activity relied largely on the acidic pH. [...] Further study of the low-pH-independent antiviral mechanism and attempts to enhance the antiviral activity may establish a novel anti-IAV therapy and vaccination strategy.*" [80]

k. Online Dossier of Scientific Research Findings:

https://theantiviraldiet.com/ingredient-%2342-%2B-research

GASTRO-MODULATORS

ALTHOUGH THIS TERM may not have been used elsewhere, I hope that it adequately describes the wide range of ingredients found under this rubric. Realizing that these dietary elements affect gastro-intestinal processes *in diverse ways* - but that this was nonetheless their uniting characteristic - I decided to bring them together under this general heading. In **Part 1**, several studies were cited which confirmed that the difference between whether a country consumed fermented food or not had a firm statistical relationship with indicence of COVID-19. Gut health is gradually being taken more seriously as a crucial determinant of a person's likelihood to contract an illness. It appears that the 'Gut Flora' or 'Gut Microbiota' - which are the microörganisms that live in our digestive tracts, including bacteria, archaea and fungi - are vital to overall state of health. Although additional research needs to be undertaken regarding each of the ingredients in this sub-section - as the preliminary findings are so significant - it seems to be established now, as a scientific fact, that a healthy gut makes a key contribution to our remaining in a better state of general health.

Fermented Food is, of all the ingredients here, the one on which we have most precise results. When food is fermented, it goes through a natural process where microörganisms (such as yeast and bacteria) convert carbohydrates (like starch and sugar) into alcohol or acids. These latter then act as a natural preservative. They are what give a zesty and tart taste to fermented food. This process preserves the food and promotes the growth of 'good bacteria' - known as probiotics - which positively impact digestion, heart health and immunity. Foods like sauerkraut, yoghurt and kombucha are fermented.

Even though honey in general is well evidenced to have a wide variety of health benefits, *Manuka Honey* has been particularly researched because of the presence of a special active ingredient called Methylglyoxal. This honey is only produced by bees who pollinate the Manuka bush (*Leptospermum Scoparium*) in New Zealand. Research has identified anti-bacterial, anti-inflammatory and antioxidant benefits in this honey. It is known for alleviating digestive issues, stopping tooth decay and soothing cold symptoms (cough, sore throat).

Spirulina, a form of 'Cyanobacteria' (blue-green algae) that is edible by humans, has been under the microscope recently in terms of its numerous reputed health benefits. It was a food source for the Aztecs and Meso-Americans but is now cultivated worldwide and sold as a dietary supplement. It appears to have potent antioxidant, anti-inflammatory and gut-health promoting qualities. It is a food-stuff high in nutrients.

Olive Leaf and Oil are both under intensive research as preliminary findings show that they are able to lower cholesterol, decrease blood pressure and prevent heart disease. In the case of Olive Leaf extract, for example - due to successful results in animals - human trials are now being conducted. It appears to be the polyphenols, such as Oleacein and Oleuropein, that are largely responsible for these health benefits.

Maitake is one of a large number of medicinal mushrooms, prized in China and surrounding regions. β-Glucans, which have already been included (*qv.* 'Nutrients') are a type of Polysaccharide - long-chain of carbohydrates - that positively affects the digestive system, immune system and more. Maitake is being researched for its ability to treat diabetes, decrease blood pressure and high cholesterol, decrease insulin resistance, as well as its multiple anti-cancer qualities.

Reishi - known as the 'Mushroom of Immortality' - has been investigated for many years as its traditional medicinal properties do appear to be supported by scientific evidence. Also known as 'Ganoderma Lucidum', the triterpenoids, polysaccharides and peptidoglycans of this fungus appear to be responsible for helping the body fight infection (including cancer cells) decreasing inflammation and aiding digestion.

These 'Gastromodulators' all have anti-viral effects.

149

Ingredient #43 FERMENTED FOOD

a. 'Fermentation' is:

*When Sugars and other Carbohydrates are converted into Alcohol **or** Preservative Organic Acids and CO_2*

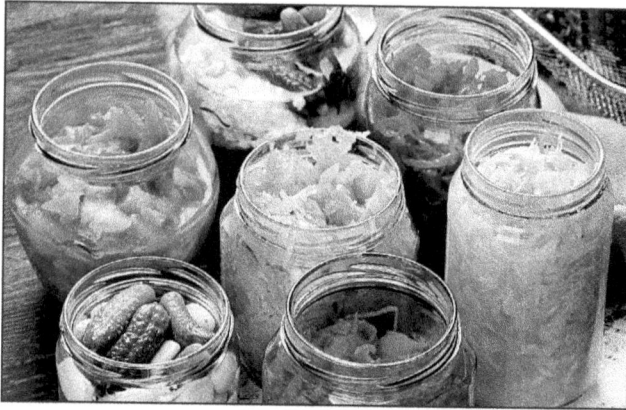

b. Fermented Items Include:

Tempeh, Kefir, Miso, Natto, Kombucha, Kimchi, Pu Erh Tea, Sauerkraut and Probiotic Yoghurts

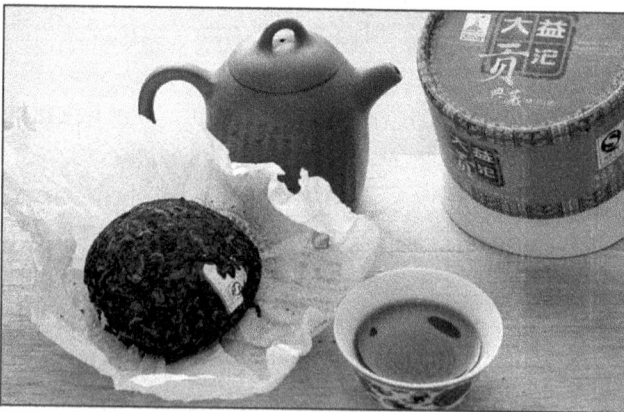

c. Not Forgetting:

Vinegars, of course - above all Traditional Cider Vinegar

d. Effect upon Viruses:
Anti-Viral Action of Fermented Foods/Drinks against Viruses is too wide an area to summarize, but they have effects against Enteroviruses, Diarrhoea Viruses *inter alia*

e. Impact on Immunity:
Friendly Bacteria in the Gut stimulate the Immune System
Deprivation of Fermented Food in Diet impacts Health

f. Additional Information:
Fermented Food in Diet may lower a Nation's Mortality Rate
It is currently being researched **re**: SARS-CoV-2 Virus

g. Recommended Daily Intake: Not Applicable

h. Human Safety: Safe at Normal Dietary Levels

i. Research Quote - Reducing COVID-19 Symptoms:
"Different levels of evidence support the use of fermented foods, probiotics and prebiotics to promote gut and lungs immunity. Without being a promise of efficacy against COVID-19, incorporating them into the diet may help to low down gut inflammation and to enhance mucosal immunity, to possibly better face the infection by contributing to diminishing the severity or the duration of infection episodes." [81]

j. Research Quote - Potential against COVID-19:
"Fermented vegetables contain many lactobacilli, which are also potent Nrf2 activators. Three examples are given: Kimchi in Korea, westernized foods and the slum paradox. It is proposed that fermented cabbage is a proof-of-concept of dietary manipulations that may enhance Nrf2-associated antioxidant effects helpful in mitigating COVID-19 severity." [82]

k. Online Dossier of Scientific Research Findings:
https://theantiviraldiet.com/ingredient-%2343-%2B-research

Ingredient #44 MĀNUKA HONEY

a. <u>Known for</u>:

*Coming only from the Nectar of the Mānuka Tree (**Leptospermum Scoparium**) native to New Zealand*

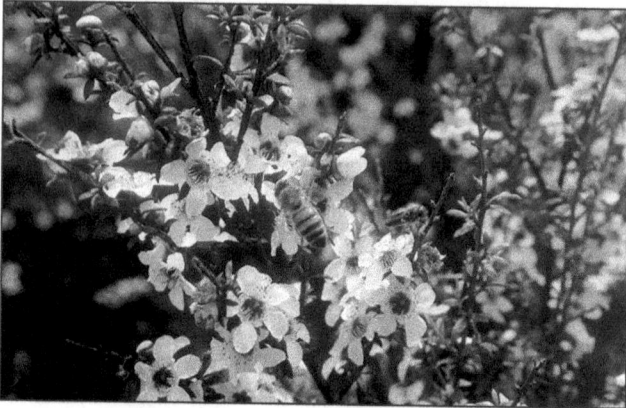

b. <u>Must be Proven to Have</u>:

Methylglyoxal (MGO), Dihydroxyacetone (DHA) to Correct Standard + DNA of Leptospermum Scoparium

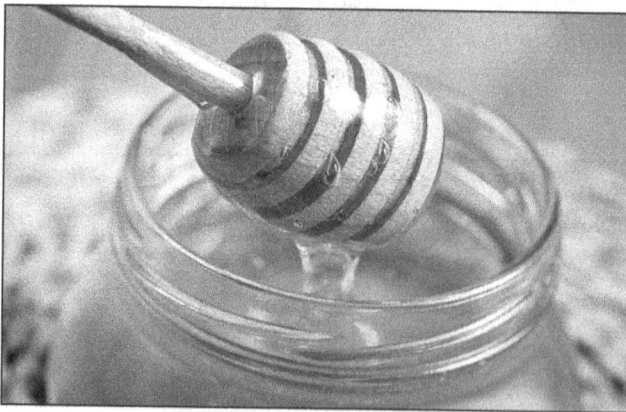

c. <u>Beware of</u>:

Counterfeit and Substandard Mānuka Honey Products

d. Effect upon Viruses:
Anti-Viral Action evidenced against Varicella Zoster Virus (which causes Chickenpox & Shingles), Adenoviruses, Influenza Viruses, Herpes Simplex Viruses, Human Immunodeficiency Virus (HIV-1) *inter alia*

e. Impact on Immunity:
Appears to stimulate Immune System Response as well

f. Additional Information:
Also Anti-Inflammatory, Antioxidant and Bactericidal. It is currently being researched **re**: SARS-CoV-2 Virus

g. Recommended Daily Intake: Not Applicable

h. Human Safety: Safe at Normal Dietary Levels

i. Research Quote - Anti-Viral against SARS-CoV-2:
"The presented study screened in silico the biological activity of six compounds present in honeybee and propolis as antiviral components against the COVID-19 main protease. The study revealed that four compounds have strong binding affinity with good glide score and may inhibit the COVID-19 main protease and virus replication." [83]

j. Research Quote - Potential against COVID-19:
"Honey can be beneficial for patients with COVID-19 caused by an enveloped virus SARS-CoV-2 through simultaneously boosting the host immune system, improving comorbid conditions and antiviral activities. Moreover, a clinical trial of honey on COVID-19 patients has been undergoing. In this review, we summarized the potential benefits of honey and its ingredients in the context of antimicrobial activities, numerous chronic diseases, and host immune system and thereby tried to establish a relationship with honey for the treatment of COVID-19." [84]

k. Online Dossier of Scientific Research Findings:
https://theantiviraldiet.com/ingredient-%2344-%2B-research

Ingredient #45 SPIRULINA

a. Found as:

Arthrospira Platensis and *Arthospira Maxima* - two types of Blue-Green Algae or 'Cyanobacteria'

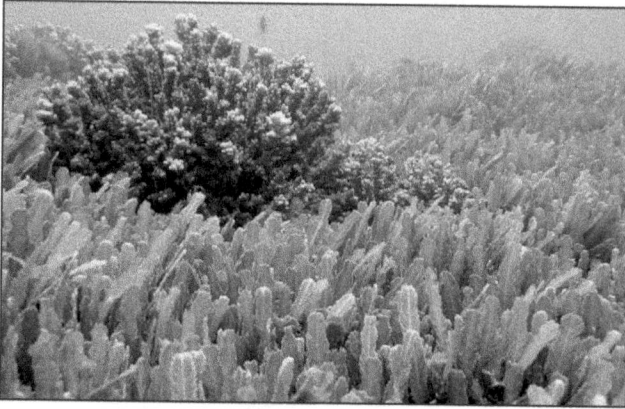

b. Available as:

A Dietary Supplement in Tablet Form and as a Whole Food in Powder Form to Combine with Foods or Drinks

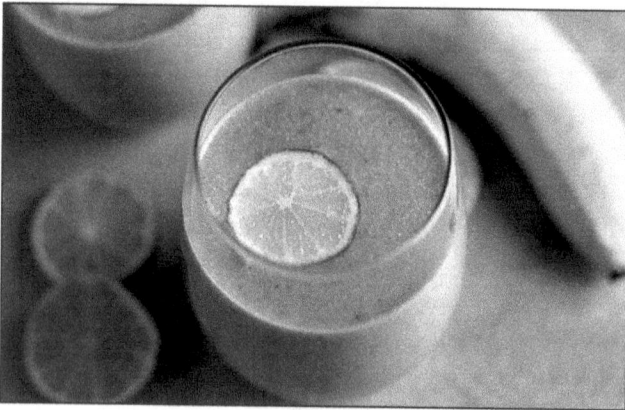

c. Amazing to Know:

Spirulina has been used by NASA Astronauts in Space

d. Effect upon Viruses:

Anti-Viral Action evidenced against Influenza Viruses, Herpes Simplex Virus Type 2, Several Coronaviruses: SARS-CoV-1, MERS-CoV & SARS-CoV-2 [in vitro]

e. Impact on Immunity:

Promotes Proliferation of Antibodies and Lymphocytes - Although Bacterial itself, it exerts Antibacterial Effects

f. Additional Information:

Also Anti-Inflammatory, Antioxidant and Anti-Allergic. It is currently being researched **re:** SARS-CoV-2 Virus

g. Recommended Daily Intake: Not Applicable

h. Human Safety: Non-Toxic but Excess can be harmful

i. Research Quote - Immuno-Modulatory Effects:

"*Spirulina is highly nutritious and has hypolipidemic, hypoglycemic and antihypertensive properties. Spirulina contains several bioactive compounds, such as phenols, phycobiliproteins and sulphated polysaccharides and many more with proven antioxidant, anti-inflammatory and immunostimulant/ immunomodulatory effects.*" [85]

j. Research Quote - Anti-Viral against COVID-19:

"*[T]he microalgal species Arthrospira platensis is high in amino acids and vitamins which help in the improvement of immunity power in human beings hence this potentiality can be utilized to fight against novel coronavirus COVID-19. This particular algal species has both immunity improving capacity and also capable of suppressing the viral activities in humans. So this alga can be recommended to use against this pandemic viral infection as a preventive remedy.*" [86]

k. Online Dossier of Scientific Research Findings:

https://theantiviraldiet.com/ingredient-%2345-%2B-research

Ingredient #46 OLIVE/LEAF & OIL

a. Taken from:

The Tree **Olea Europaea** - the Active Ingredient **Oleuropein** is found in both the Leaves and Fruit

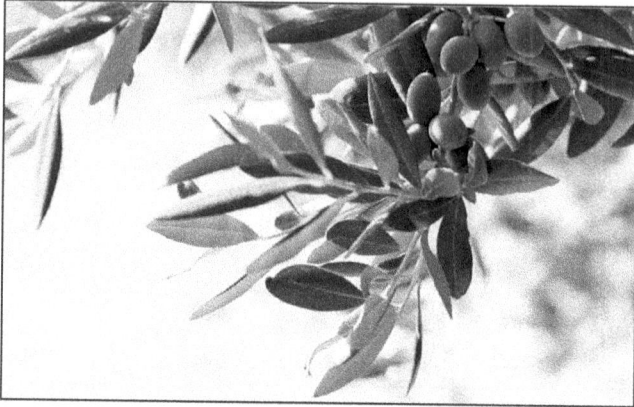

b. Available in:

Olives, Olive Oil and Olive Leaf Extract. Recorded use of the Oil within Ancient Israelite Cuisine is in the Bible

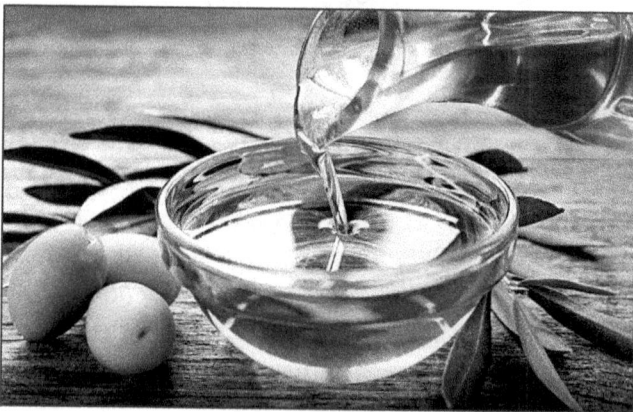

c. Amazing to Know:

Some Olive Trees still living are over 2000 Years Old

d. Effect upon Viruses:
Anti-Viral Action evidenced against Newcastle Disease Virus, Influenza, Rotaviruses, Hepatitis Viruses, Herpes Simplex Viruses, Human Syncytial Virus, Parainfluenza Type 3, Viral Hemorrhagic Septicemia Virus, Human Immunodeficiency Virus (HIV-1) *inter alia.*

e. Impact on Immunity:
Main Impact of Oleuropein is Direct Anti-Viral Action *qv.* d.

f. Additional Information:
Also Anti-Inflammatory, Antioxidant and Anti-Allergic. It is currently being researched **re:** SARS-CoV-2 Virus

g. Recommended Daily Intake: Not Applicable

h. Human Safety: Safe at Normal Dietary Levels

i. Research Quote - Anti-Viral against SARS-CoV-2:
"*Therefore, nelfinavir and lopinavir may represent potential treatment options, and kaempferol, quercetin, luteolin-7-gluco-side, demethoxycurcumin, naringenin, apigenin-7-glucoside, oleuropein, curcumin, catechin, and epicatechin-gallate appeared to have the best potential to act as COVID-19 Mpro inhibitors. However, further research is necessary to investigate their potential medicinal use.*" [87]

j. Research Quote - Oleuropein as Anti-Viral:
"*Many studies have shown that OLE [Oleuropein] possesses a strong antioxidative activity but this property does not seem directly related to its antiviral effect. The results indicate that O. europaea crude extract can be considered as a potential source of anti-Newcastle virus agent by its effect on viral gene expression. The effects are comparable with IFN-β which is known antiviral cytokine of the host.*" [88]

k. Online Dossier of Scientific Research Findings:
https://theantiviraldiet.com/ingredient-%2346-%2B-research

Ingredient #47 MAITAKE

a. Known as:

Grifola Frondosa or 'Hen-of-the-Woods' - though the Japanese name is 舞茸 or 'Dancing Mushroom'

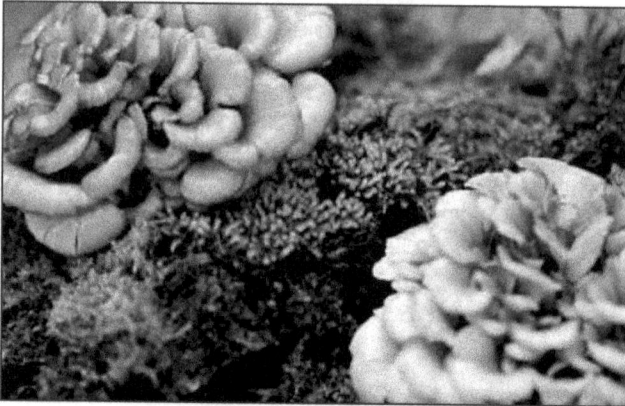

b. Available as:

Fresh Mushrooms, Dessicated Mushrooms, Maitake Mushroom Powder & Maitake D-Fraction Supplement

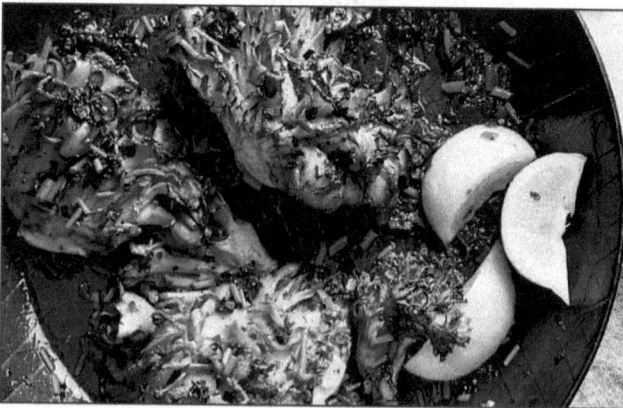

c. Worth Knowing:

Typically grows at the base of Elms, Oak & Maple Trees

d. Effect upon Viruses:
Indirectly, by Stimulation of the Immune System qv. **e.**

e. Impact on Immunity:
Glucan Polysaccharides in Maitake have an Immuno-modulatory Effect on the Immune System, both Humoral Immunity (including Antibodies) and Cell Immunity (Blood). Production of Cytokines IL-6, IL-12 and IFN-γ is enhanced.

f. Additional Information:
Also Anti-Inflammatory, Antioxidant and Bactericidal. It is currently being researched **re:** SARS-CoV-2 Virus

g. Recommended Daily Intake: Not Applicable

h. Human Safety: Safe at Normal Dietary Levels

i. Research Quote - Immuno-Modulatory Agent:
"Here, we made a brief review of the current findings on fungi as producers of protease inhibitors and studies on the relevant candidate fungal bioactive compounds that can offer immunomodulatory activities as potential therapeutic agents of coronaviruses in the future." [89]

j. Research Quote - Anti-Bacterial and Anti-Viral:
"In this clinical trial, we demonstrated that Maitake intake enhanced antibody production in response to influenza vaccination while simultaneously suppressing multiple common cold symptoms. The current results suggest that Maitake may activate both innate and adaptive immune responses for the prevention of virus infection. In conclusion, we expect that Maitake intake potentiates host defense systems and has a protective effect against influenza virus and other pathogenic viruses and bacteria." [90]

k. Online Dossier of Scientific Research Findings:
https://theantiviraldiet.com/ingredient-%2347-%2B-research

Ingredient #48 REISHI

a. Known as:

Ganoderma Lingzhi or *Ganoderma Lingzhi* - for its health benefits, as the 'Mushroom of Immortality'

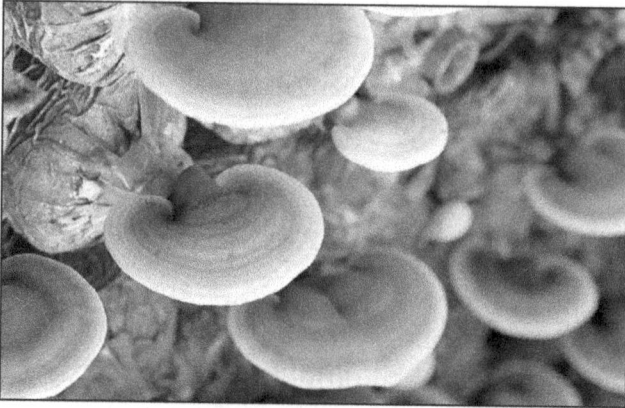

b. Available as:

Whole Mushrooms, in Dessicated Form or as a Bitter Powder Extract - for example within 'Lingzhi Coffee'

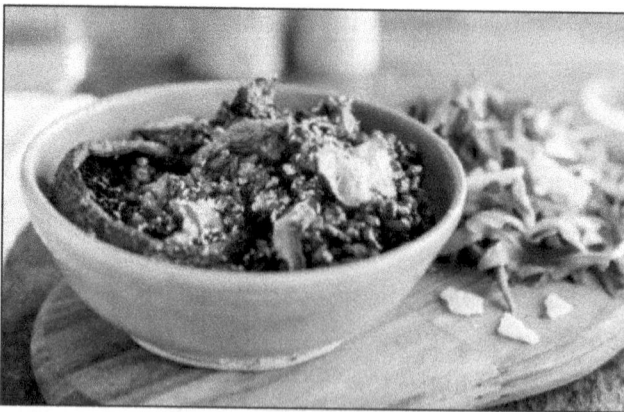

c. Historically:

Reishi Mushroom's Use is recorded in the 1st Century CE

d. Effect upon Viruses:
Anti-Viral Action evidenced against Dengue Fever Virus Type 2, Herpes Simplex Viruses, Enterovirus-71 *inter alia*.

e. Impact on Immunity:
Glucan Polysaccharides in Maitake have an Immuno-modulatory Effect on the Immune System, both Humoral Immunity (including Antibodies) and Cell Immunity (Blood).

f. Additional Information:
Also Anti-Inflammatory, Antioxidant and Bactericidal. It is currently being researched **re:** SARS-CoV-2 Virus

g. Recommended Daily Intake: Not Applicable

h. Human Safety: Safe at Normal Dietary Levels

i. Research Quote - Immuno-Modulatory Effect:
"An early study highlighted that the anti-inflammatory and NRF2-inducer potencies of 18 triterpenoids correlated linearly over six orders of magnitude of concentration, suggesting that the two processes are mechanistically linked. Some triterpenoids isolated from Ganoderma lucidum have been found to be potential inhibitors of the NS2B-NS3 protease of DENV." [91]

j. Research Quote - Effect upon SARS-CoV-2:
"Studies from different countries have shown that polysaccharides, as well as other fungal compounds (nucleosides, proteins, terpenoids, glycoproteins, etc.) exert antiviral effect against many viruses pathogenic for humans such as orthopoxviruses, herpes, hepatitis viruses, West Nile, human immunodeficiency, and influenza. Biologically active compounds prepared from the same fungal species can show antiviral activities against different viral pathogens." [92]

k. Online Dossier of Scientific Research Findings:
https://theantiviraldiet.com/ingredient-%2348-%2B-research

OTHER PHYTOCHEMICALS

ALTHOUGH THE INGREDIENTS *here* find themselves in a section which may have the appearance of being 'miscellaneous', I was unable to make a firm decision on where else to best place them. In three cases, we are dealing with isolated compounds that occur in a variety of food sources, whereas in one case what we have is a natural ingredient which contains a number of bioactive compounds. A uniting characteristic of the four ingredients featured here, is that in all four cases we are concerned with chemicals derived from plants, not occurring in meats or other sources – so *phytochemicals*.

Even though a small number of ingredients in this antiviral diet do occur at a greater level in meats and fish, every ingredient can also be found in a plant source of some kind. As emphasized in the opening stage of this book, this is neither a vegetarian nor meat-eater's diet, but can be customized according to your preferences and beliefs. As for the four ingredients in this sub-section, none of them could be excluded as the evidence in favour of their anti-viral effects and/or immune supportive properties is already of a sufficient kind. Like before, let us take a look at each of these ingredients briefly.

Resveratrol, possessed of the daunting chemical name 3,5,4′-trihydroxy-trans-stilbene, is also from the broad family of natural phenols, to which the flavonoids (*qv.*) belong. It is a chemical that is produced by plants when being attacked by pathogens – bacteria, viruses *et alia* – or in response to an injury of some kind. Sources of resveratrol include grapes (in particular the skin), mulberries, raspberries and even peanuts. Resveratrol has a large body of evidence behind its anti-bacterial, fungicidal, anti-inflammatory and cancer-preventive properties. Its potential continues to be researched intensely.

Sambucus Nigra is the proper name for the Elderberry, a fruit which has traditionally been credited with having many medicinal properties. It is a plant rich in many nutrients – proteins, carbohydrates, fats, minerals, vitamins, essential oils *et al.* – but also (like Resveratrol) contains some natural polyphenols which are responsible for its anti-oxidative, anti-inflammatory, anti-bacterial and anti-viral qualities. Both the leaves and fruit contain therapeutic ingredients and Sambucus Nigra is being researched more deeply due to its anti-SARS-CoV-2 effects.

d-Limonene, also simply known as 'Limonene', is one of the essential oils found in the peel of lemons and other citrus fruits. It has been extracted from these fruits for centuries and used as a natural remedy for a number of health issues. Now, most typically, you will find it in a great many products to give them a pleasant taste or scent. However, although it is most concentrated in the peel (of the orange, especially), it is present in far smaller amounts in the fruit and juices taken from them. Limonene is from the family of terpenes, whose strong smell will deter parasites and other threats. This terpene is well evidenced as having anti-inflammatory, antioxidant, anti-bacterial, anti-fungal and anti-infective qualities.

Anethole, perhaps the most bioactive ingredient in star anise and fennel – both of which have long been prized for their medicinal properties – was first extracted from them by the German alchemist Hieronymus Brunschwig in the 15th century. Anethole, also known as 'Anise Camphor' is what gives several foods the inimitable taste we recognize as aniseed. This phytochemical is evidenced to have potent bactericidal, fungicidal, anti-inflammatory and antioxidant properties.

It is important to reiterate that the fifty-two ingredients presented in this section overall are not intended as a 'be all and end all' list of what should be the ingredients of an anti-viral diet. They are only a starting list. Even though I have attempted to make this base-list as well-founded on research and as well-evidenced in their anti-viral qualities as possible, **AVD** is a work in progress, whose adjustment in line with new scientific findings is the best way that it will come to maturity.

163

Ingredient #49 RESVERATROL

a. <u>Richly Found in</u>:
Red Grape Juice, Red Grapes, Blueberries, Bilberries, Cranberries, Peanuts & Cocoa

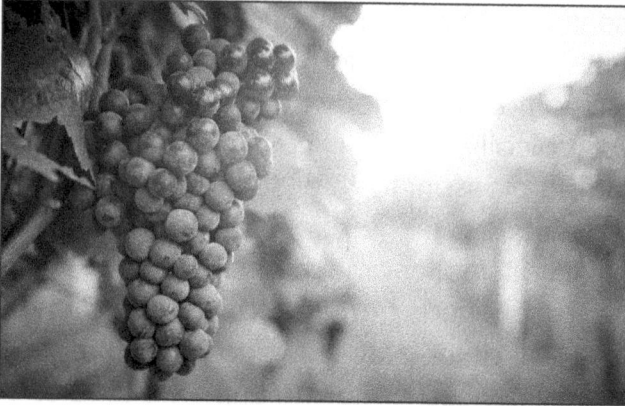

b. <u>Other Sources include</u>:
Peanut-Butter, Pistachios, Dark Chocolate, Milk Chocolate, Strawberries & Red Wine

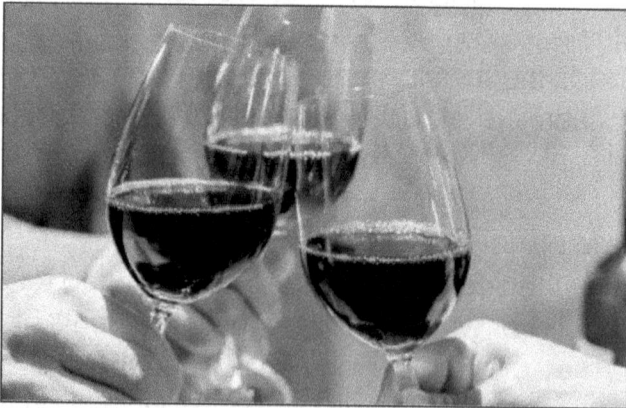

c. <u>Worth Knowing</u>:
Red Wines from Madiran are the Richest in Resveratrol

d. Effect upon Viruses:
Anti-Viral Action evidenced against Varicella Zoster Virus, Cytomegalovirus, Influenza A Virus, Polyomavirus, Hepatitis C Virus, Respiratory Syncytial Virus, Epstein-Barr Virus, HIV, Herpes Simplex Virus 1 & 2, Human Rhinovirus, Human Metapneumonia Virus, Enterovirus-71, HCV, MERS-CoV

e. Impact on Immunity:
In Low Doses Resveratrol stimulates the Immune System

f. Additional Information:
Also Anti-Inflammatory, Antioxidant and Bactericidal

g. Recommended Daily Intake: Not Applicable

h. Human Safety: Safe at Normal Dietary Levels

i. Research Quote - Immuno-Modulatory Effect:
"*Based on the results, we report that stilbene based compounds in general and resveratrol, in particular, can be promising anti-COVID-19 drug candidates acting through disruption of the spike protein. Our findings in this study are promising and call for further in vitro and in vivo testing of stilbenoids, especially resveratrol against the COVID-19.*" [93]

j. Research Quote - Effect upon SARS-CoV-2:
"*Resveratrol has been reported to exhibit antiviral properties against a variety of viral pathogens in vitro and in vivo. [...] Although there are no data for using resveratrol in humans infected with SARS-CoV-2, the above studies demonstrate that this compound may be an adjunctive antiviral agent to consider, especially based on the data published by Linn et al showing activity against MERS-CoV in vitro. Although dosing in humans is unknown, resveratrol is considered safe when taken at supplemental doses.*" [94]

k. Online Dossier of Scientific Research Findings:
https://theantiviraldiet.com/ingredient-%2349-%2B-research

Ingredient #50 ELDERBERRY

a. Known as:

Sambucus Nigra - from the plant family the Adoxaceae - is also known as 'European Elderberry' & 'Black Elder'

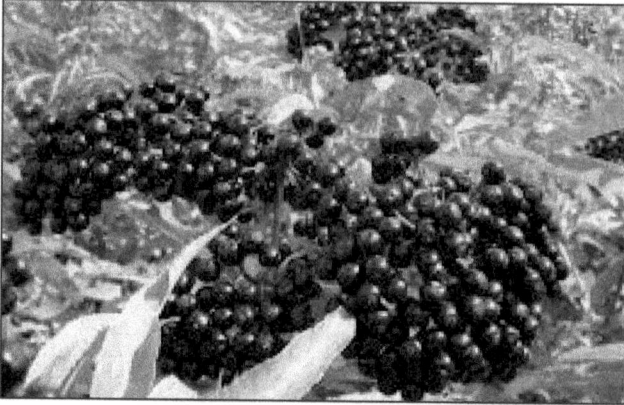

b. Available as:

Fresh Berries - but should be cooked to be eaten. Also made into Juice, Preserve, Chutney, Wine and in Pies

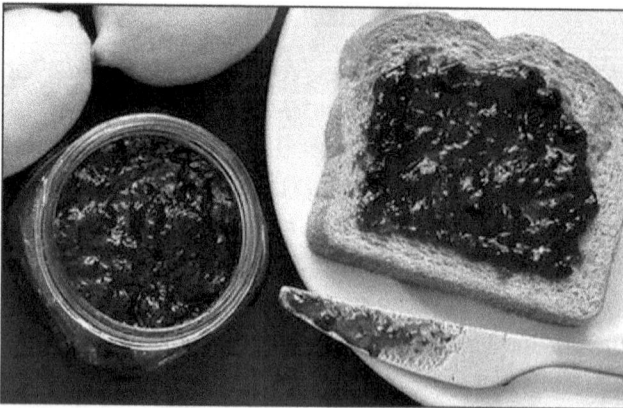

c. Also Available as:

Lozenges, Syrups & Capsules - to treat Cold Symptoms

d. Effect upon Viruses:
Anti-Viral Action evidenced against Influenza A Virus, Influenza B Virus, Influenza H1N1 Virus, Infectious Bronchitis Virus, Human Immunodeficiency Virus (HIV-1)

e. Impact on Immunity:
Main Impact of Sambucus is Direct Anti-Viral Action *qv.* **d.**

f. Additional Information:
Also Anti-Inflammatory, Antioxidant and Bactericidal. It is currently being researched **re:** SARS-CoV-2 Virus – deemed promising as it affects other Envelope Viruses

g. Recommended Daily Intake: Not Applicable

h. Human Safety: Uncooked Elderberries can be Toxic

i. Research Quote – Immuno-Modulatory Effect:
"The S. nigra inactivates two distinct envelope viruses and should be tested on Ebola, also an envelope virus, as it is likely that it may inactivate that too. It should also be tested on SARS and other novel coronaviruses such as COVID-19 which are all envelope viruses. Other species of Sambucus appear to have very similar properties including inhibiting coronaviruses. Elderberry seems to have potential as a useful medicine, particularly since there are reasons to believe resistance to it is unlikely to ever develop." [95]

j. Research Quote – Effect upon SARS-CoV-2:
"Given the body of evidence from preclinical studies demonstrating the antiviral effects of S.nigra berry, alongside the results from clinical studies involving influenza viral infections included in this review, pre-clinical research exploring the potential effects of S.nigra berry on COVID-19 are encouraged." [96]

k. Online Dossier of Scientific Research Findings:
https://theantiviraldiet.com/ingredient-%2350-%2B-research

Ingredient #51 LIMONENE

a. Richly Found in:

Lemons, Oranges, Limes, Grapefruit & Mandarins
(it is most concentrated in the peel of the fruit)

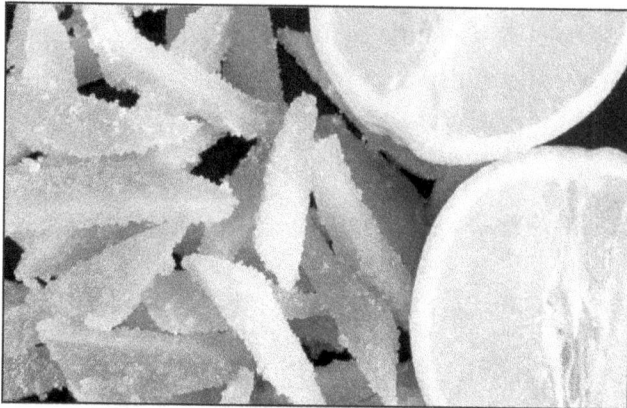

b. However, Be Aware that:

Many Foods/Drinks have Limonene Added to them –
Only Naturally Occurring Limonene is Recommended

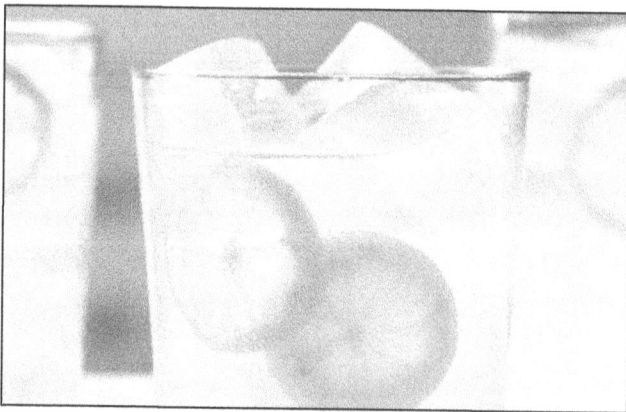

c. Suggestion:

A Slice of Fruit in your Drink will add some Limonene to it

d. Effect upon Viruses:

Anti-Viral Action evidenced against Yellow Fever Virus, Herpes Simplex Virus Type 1, Influenza Viruses, Coronavirus SARS-CoV-1 *inter alia*

e. Impact on Immunity:

Main Impact of Limonene is Direct Anti-Viral Action *qv.* d. Causes Proliferation of Antibodies & White Blood Cells

f. Additional Information:

Also Anti-Inflammatory, Antioxidant and Bactericidal. It is currently being researched **re**: SARS-CoV-2 Virus

g. Recommended Daily Intake: Not Applicable

h. Human Safety: Non-Toxic but Excess can be harmful

i. Research Quote – Immuno-Modulatory Effect:

"Next, we found that treatment with citronellol and limonene significantly downregulated ACE2 expression in epithelial cells. The results suggest that geranium and lemon essential oils and their derivative compounds are valuable natural anti-viral agents that may contribute to the prevention of the invasion of SARS-CoV-2/COVID-19 into the human body." [97]

j. Research Quote – Effect upon SARS-CoV-2:

"The maximum total WBC count in carvone treated animals was observed on the 12th day (16,560 cells/cmm) while in limonene (13,783 cells/cmm) and perillic acid (14,437 cells/cmm) treated animals the maximum count was observed on the 9th day after the drug treatment. Administration of terpenoids increased the total antibody production, antibody producing cells in spleen, bone marrow cellularity and alpha-esterase positive cells significantly compared to the normal animals indicating its potentiating effect on the immune system." [98]

k. Online Dossier of Scientific Research Findings:

https://theantiviraldiet.com/ingredient-%2351-%2B-research

Ingredient #52 ANETHOLE

a. <u>Richly Found in</u>:

*Anise, Star Anise, Fennel, Anise Myrtle,
Liquorice, Camphor & Magnolia Blossom*

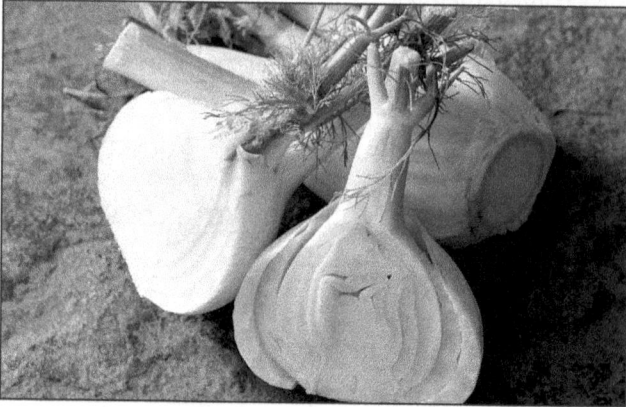

b. <u>Also Present in</u>:

*Peppermints, Wild Celeries & Coriander; also in
Nutmegs, Cumins, Lemon Balms & Common Thyme*

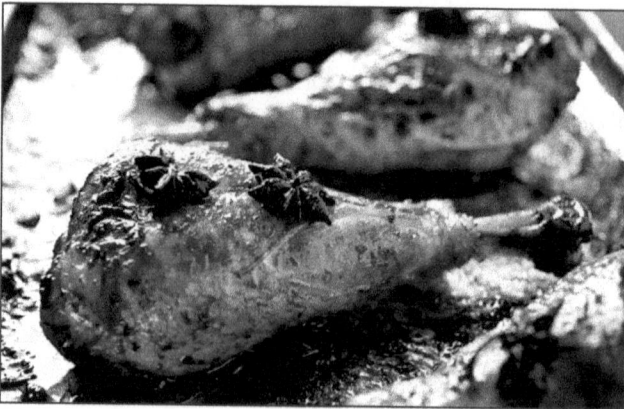

c. <u>Recognizable</u>:

By the Inimitable Taste of Aniseed in Foods and Drinks

170

d. Effect upon Viruses:
Anti-Viral Action evidenced against Herpes Simplex Virus Type 1, Herpes Simplex Virus Type 2, Para-influenza Virus Type 3 *inter alia*

e. Impact on Immunity:
Main Impact of Anethole is Direct Anti-Viral Action *qv.* d. Also Immunomodulatory *viz.* Regulation of Cytokines

f. Additional Information:
Also Anti-Inflammatory, Antioxidant and Bactericidal. It is currently being researched **re:** SARS-CoV-2 Virus

g. Recommended Daily Intake: Not Applicable

h. Human Safety: Safe at Normal Dietary Levels

i. Research Quote - Immuno-Modulatory Effect:
"*Our data showed that trans-anethole and estragole promote some changes in the immune system by reducing the delayed-type hypersensitivity response, and increasing the number of leucocytes in peripheral blood in mice. Also, we observed that trans-anethole improved the humoral response.*" [99]

j. Research Quote - Effect upon SARS-CoV-2:
"*Illicium verum essential oil inhibited viral infectivity by 99%, while phenylpropanoids reduced the HSV infectivity by 60–80% and sesquiterpenes inhibited the infectivity by 40–98%. In another study, anise oil showed dose-dependent antiviral activity against HSV-2. There was no inhibitory effect when the essential oils were added to the cells before infection or after the adsorption period. The authors concluded that essential oils may interact with the virus envelope and prevent the adsorption of the virus.*" [100]

k. Online Dossier of Scientific Research Findings:
https://theantiviraldiet.com/ingredient-%2352-%2B-research

PART 2   THE ANTI-VIRAL DIET
KEY POINTS

1. *Guidelines of the World Health Organization on Dietary Intake and Recommendations regarding a Balanced Diet, are Base Guidelines for this Anti-Viral Diet*

2. *There are Numerous Dietary Hazards to Avoid for Viral Protection - including High Fat & Sugar Intake, Alcohol, Smoking & Recreational Drugs*

3. *This Part of the Anti-Viral Diet presents 52 Ingredients that Current Scientific Evidence corroborates as having Anti-Viral Properties*

4. *Some of these Ingredients have Direct or Indirect Effects upon Viruses and Viral Illnesses*

5. *Other of these Ingredients have Various Types of Effect on the Human Immune System*

6. *Both Types of Ingredients - both those with Anti-Viral Effects and those with Immunomodulatory Qualities - **may help** to protect you from Viruses and Viral Illnesses*

7. *Vitamins are the 1*st *Group of Ingredients that can exert Anti-Viral Effects - mainly through supporting the Immune System*

8. *Minerals are the 2*nd *Group of Ingredients that can exert Anti-Viral Effects - also mainly through support of the Immune System*

9. *There are Other Nutrients that can exert Anti-Viral Effects, some through Inhibiting Viruses and others by Optimizing the Effectiveness of the Immune System*

10. *The Flavonoids can exert Anti-Viral Effects - mainly through Inhibition of the Replication of Viruses*

11. *A Number of Herbs and Spices - some used in Traditional Medicine - have an Effect on the Immune System or may directly Inhibit Viruses*

12. *A Number of Plants and Flowers - used in Teas and Beverages and TCM - have Anti-Viral and Immune System Effects*

13. *Several Compounds have Special Impact on the Gut, exerting Anti-Viral and Immuno-Enhancing Effects*

14. *The Anti-Viral Diet continues to seek out New Anti-Viral Ingredients, on the Basis of Scientific Evidence*

PART 3
CREATING YOUR DIET

CREATING YOUR DIET

11. SELECTING YOUR INGREDIENTS

YOU HAVE JUST LEARNT what the core ingredients of **AVD** are - for the time being. I have not compiled that dossier of 52 ingredients so as to tell you that you *must* use all of them. Rather, I have provided data on *those* dietary elements and not others, because they are the ones for which a significant amount of research findings already exist in regard to their anti-viral qualities or immuno-supportive properties. Others will be added - with equal or greater evidence behind them - but I just wish to emphasize that this has remained the test throughout this diet: that sufficient scientific corroboration exists, which either proves or at the very least is powerfully indicative of anti-viral attributes being applied to an ingredient.

I have used the terms 'dietary element' and 'ingredient' quite interchangeably in this book - not out of a spirit of vagueness or confusion, but because the substances I am referring to are both of those things at the same time. The foods and plants and compounds included here are being proposed as possible *elements* of your anti-viral diet. At the same time - when it comes to preparing food - we refer to the many different items as *ingredients* - which also indicates that they are going to be combined with other food. I need to reiterate here, that just because countless ingredients are not listed in this book, does not mean that they should be avoided. As will be explained more clearly in a moment, the idea of an anti-viral diet is not that every ingredient one eats must have an anti-viral or immune supportive property. That would be excessive and unnecessary. The general idea of such a diet is simply to *increase* the quantity of ingredients you eat which may be capable of protecting you from viruses and strengthen your immune system. The entire supermarket of ingredients is still at your disposal - don't worry about that.

I don't have anything complicated to explain in **Part 3** of this book. The scientists and medical researchers, in all honesty, have done the difficult and complex work that was needed - over a long period of time - in order to arrive at the possibility of this prototype for an anti-viral diet. However, as "*common sense isn't all that common*", like the saying goes, it is vital that I do give *some* words of explanation and guidance here, so that the purpose of this book is not misunderstood.

I am not going to create a body of rules or regulations, or some strict dietary codes to follow. What is provided in this book is just the *basis* of an anti-viral diet in the broadest sense and not a strict regimen of what you must eat - and how, and when - as is the case in numerous diets that I have surveyed. There is no point in my producing any artificial rules that are more likely going to put people off from engaging with this diet. What I will provide, however, especially in **Section 14** of this part, is some down-to-earth advice on how you can make **AVD** work for you, in the simplest way possible. That chapter explains the key principle of the 'Anti-Viral 5-a-Day'.

Even if you have not read **Part 1** of this book, and have only perhaps glanced through the ingredients in **Part 2**, it is still just as easy for you get started with an anti-viral diet, one that *may* offer you a significant degree of natural protection against viruses and viral illnesses. At this point in time - with no cure yet in sight for COVID-19 and still no approved vaccines available - alternative treatment options should not be cast out of mind, without consideration. What I would emphasize at this stage, even if you have not considered any evidence in support of the anti-viral ingredients included here, is that all of the dietary elements presented in the previous part of this book are known to be safe and non-toxic in normal quantities. If you were to begin consuming some of those ingredients - as part of whatever diet of food you are eating - the likelihood is that they would contribute to your being healthier on a general level, whatever your view is of their *anti-virality*.

I want you to understand that this diet is not *prescri-bing* what you should do, only *offering you some suggestions*, based on scientific findings. I have not listed the ingredients in **Part 2** so as to then say: "*These are the Viral Cures – Now Eat them and Be Well!*" The data in that selected list of in-gredients – for each of which you can find supplementary re-search dossiers online – has been provided so as to get you familiar with the properties that they appear to possess, not to dictate what you should eat. Eating, like most things in life, is based on choice, so *choice* remains at the core of this diet. However, making "informed choices" is based upon having ample information about the decisions you are making, and that is why a considerable amount of information has been provided on the anti-viral ingredients being proposed here.

In my opinion, once chemicals – occurring in foodstuffs – have been shown to have anti-viral effects *in vitro*, perhaps *in vivo* too, and much evidence points toward anti-viral pro-perties being confirmed, I do not think it is necessary to wait for clinical trials before deciding whether to include those natural chemicals in one's own diet. This is where freedom of choice is the determining factor, for the final choice is always yours.

Right now, what I would like you to do, is to review the ingredients in **Part 2** of this book and consider which ones you would like to include in your daily diet. If you know, of course, that you consume one of these dietary elements on a day-to-day basis already – and you are happy continuing – then that can of course be included. What I would especially like you to do, is to think about which *new* ingredients you would be willing to give a try, if only for a 'trial period'. Once you have looked over all of the ingredients, choose twenty that you will identify as your 'Top 20 Anti-Viral Ingredients' for now. In each case, you can write the name of a food that contains that ingredient, or name of the exact ingredient given in **Part 2**. There is a space on the next two pages for you to write up your list of twenty chosen ingredients. – *I will leave you to it.*

MY TOP TWENTY ANTI-VIRAL INGREDIENTS :

1.

2.

3.

4.

5.

6.

7.

8.

9.

10.

Not including an ingredient here does not exclude it from your **AVD**
This list is just being created in order to ensure you have at least 20

11.

12.

13.

14.

15.

16.

17.

18.

19.

20.

12. <u>SEVERAL SAFETY PRECAUTIONS</u>

HOPEFULLY, CREATING A LIST of top twenty ingredients from those in **Part 2** will have helped you to gain some focus in terms of how <u>AVD</u> could be made to work for you. The point is not to limit your diet to twenty ingredients only, but to make sure that you have at least twenty ingredients that you are ready to include in your own anti-viral diet - as a minimum.

Before proceeding any further, it is best to address some obvious issues of safety, as these cannot be ignored. A number of remarks need to be made, some of which may seem to be superfluous, but it is essential that they are said all the same.

In the *first* place, <u>AVD</u> is in no way to be treated like a 'Crash Diet'. Many of the ingredients presented in **Part 2**, if ingested in excessive quantity, can have negative effects on your health instead of just the positive ones desired. None of the ingredients have been included as a 'Virus Cure' and it would be a misunderstanding of this diet to believe that. All of the ingredients are safe to be ingested in small quantities or at the Recommended Daily Intakes - data which is easily obtained for Vitamins, Minerals and the most basic nutrients. Please be aware that some ingredients listed - for example *Sambucus Nigra* - can be lethally toxic when not cooked.

Secondly, it is essential that you make sure that you do not consume any ingredients included in the list of fifty-two if you have a food allergy or intolerance that would be affected by them. If you have a nut allergy, for example - even though Brazil nuts are one of the richest sources of the element Selenium - eating them would of course be impossible for you, in the light of your allergy. Usually, however, you will find that even though you cannot intake one of the dietary elements from one food type, it will be possible to do so from another. For example, in the case of Selenium, you might be able to gain that valuable micronutrient from Yellowfin tuna instead.

Thirdly, it is essential to bear in mind underlying health conditions when you choose to eat a dietary ingredient from the list. One of the most important factors to bear in mind is blood pressure. If an ingredient is known to lower blood pressure – and you already have a low blood pressure – then ingesting that ingredient, even in a small quantity, may create a dangerous health situation. For example, curcumin causes blood pressure to lower, so it may be advisable to avoid this spice or just try it in small quantities and see how your body reacts as a precaution. Herbs and spices are potent ingredients, and care must be taken in how they affect your body.

Fourthly, and very importantly, if you do have a health condition for which you are prescribed any form of medication, be sure to check that there are no known interactions between the ingredients you have chosen for your diet and the medicine that you take. For example, Grapefruit juice interacts with the Leukemia drug Imatinib, causing blood levels of that medication (Imatinib Mesylate) to increase to higher levels in the blood. St. John's Wort, as another example, is a herbal ingredient that interacts with numerous drugs. In case of doubt, refer to your medical practitioner and ask them if there is a chance of interaction between your medication and any of the natural ingredients you are choosing to consume.

The above are not intended as a complete list of safety precautions but just a few key issues to bear in mind when introducing new ingredients into your diet. The obvious point to state is: make sure that you are following an overall healthy balanced diet, as provided by WHO's online guidance at: www.who.int/news-room/fact-sheets/detail/healthy-diet
Also, be aware that some ingredients can have cumulative negative effects when taken in excess quantity daily, just like eating a bit too much fat daily can result in being overweight. Green tea, for example, when consumed in excess quantity – say, over eight mugs daily – can interfere with iron absorption negatively and cause Iron Deficiency Anemia.

13. <u>YOUR ANTI-VIRAL FIVE-A-DAY</u>

IT HAS TAKEN TIME, but through the initiatives and guidance of the World Health Organization - for more than seventy years and now across 150 countries worldwide - a wide public has become aware of proper nutritional guidelines as part of their general efforts to educate this planet about crucial health issues. We have come a long way since they were founded in 1948, but sadly malnutrition still affects our world badly: with an estimated 462 million adults being underweight, 144 million children (under five) being stunted, 47 million wasted and over 14 million severely wasted. Spreading more knowledge and assisting those countries where malnutrition is currently a problem, is clearly a vital task for our time, and one which all countries globally should contribute towards alleviating.

However, focusing upon the positive that *has been accomplished*, one simple working principle has found its ways into more people's lives than any other - perhaps because it has such a clear, self-descriptive title - that of '5-a-Day'. The principle is part of a drive by WHO to promote healthy eating in all countries. In their current 'Practical Advice on Maintaining a Healthy Diet', they describe the principle and two of its most direct benefits, like a simple rule-of-thumb:

"*Eating at least 400g, or five portions, of fruit and vegetables per day reduces the risk of NCDs* [non-communicable diseases] *and helps to ensure an adequate daily intake of dietary fibre.*"

It is easy to remember - easy to apply. WHO described the purpose of '5-a-Day' at their 4th International Symposium:

"*5 a day is as an international programme designed to encourage fruit and vegetable consumption, with the specific goal of encouraging all women, children and men to consume at least five servings of fruit and vegetables every day.*"

What WHO recommends is something which is so simple to put into practice that - as a result - this program has become immensely successful and had a positive impact on dozens of nations. The reality is that - because of the high presence of vitamins, minerals, flavonoids and other key nutrients across the vast range of fruit and vegetables one can choose from - by eating 'five a day' in that sense, one does go a significant distance towards protecting oneself from viral illness, especially through fortification of the immune system.

However, even though you can get a great amount of protection from illnesses through consuming a '5-a-Day' diet, this is not the only important principle to follow. Nor does WHO set this down as the sole piece of guidance in their 'Practical Advice on Maintaining a Healthy Diet' but as one of a group of straightforward dietary guidelines. For example, they also recommend that people limit their fat, salt and sugar intake at specific levels, also stressing the vital importance of breastfeeding to human health at the earliest stages of life.

The main point that this entire book is trying to share, is that even in our present state of scientific knowledge, a wide range of findings appear to indicate that there are other ingredients of great benefit, apart from fruit and vegetables. There appear to be a number of compounds - found within the flowers, root, bark and other parts of plants - that have clear actions upon viruses and the immune system. Much has also been learnt about naturally occurring chemicals in fungi and about bacteria which can have beneficial effects in our gut - as well as other ingredients, some even found in meat and organ-meat, with positive anti-viral effects. This volume has aimed to share some of the knowledge we have - of those anti-viral ingredients - in **Part 2**. The main proposal that I wish to make in this part, is that I believe it would be a beneficial principle to make a point of having at least five anti-viral ingredients on a daily basis. I will do my best to clarify this principle on the following page and answer some obvious queries.

ANTI-VIRAL FIVE-A-DAY PRINCIPLE

Having FIVE Anti-Viral Ingredients Every Day <u>may</u> Increase Your Protection against Viruses

because

(a) Some Anti-Viral Ingredients have a Direct or Indirect Inhibitory Effect on *some* Viruses

(b) Other Anti-Viral Ingredients can Enhance the Effectiveness of the Immune System

I have set out the principle of an 'Anti-Viral 5-a-Day' in the simplest way that I could in the box above. Please be assured that I am not setting this down as a scientific principle but as just one piece of practical advice which I feel confident enough to conclude from the incredible base of research that has taken place in Food Science, Nutrition, Phytochemicals, Biochemistry, Microbiology, Epidemiology, Infectious Diseases and other areas - in particular over the past fifty years.

It is a suggestion and neither a scientific conclusion nor a medical prescription. Please notice that it says that having five anti-viral ingredients every day <u>may</u> increase your protection against viruses. Just as it is impossible to predict what specific effect a medication will have on any person's body, there is no way that the author of a book - or any scientist or medical practitioner for that matter - can predict the exact dietary effect of consuming certain ingredients. At the same time, though, it is not unwarranted - based on *in vitro, in vivo* and human evidence (in some cases) – to draw some preliminary conclusions about the effects that those ingredients may have. The results of further research are awaited with great expectation, but in the light of the current dangers to which we are exposed by some fatal viruses – including SARS-CoV-2, Ebola and others – I believe there is a reasonable basis for drawing some inferences, based on probability though not certainty.

Sure, if science were to prove that any or all of the dietary elements in this book are *not* capable of offering us any protection against viruses, then I would accept those conclusions – for if something has been proven by facts, then it is true. However, with our knowledge still in a state of transformation and development, I believe that it may be down to individuals to decide what preliminary opiniond they are ready to arrive at – those, perhaps, that one may safely infer from results and analyses that have already been provided by science.

AVD only represents a personal body of reasonings that I believe may be drawn from scientific evidence existing at this time. It refers throughout to facts and results from science. The diet itself, specially this principle of an 'Anti-Viral 5-a-Day', is presented as a proposition for your consideration, not a conclusion that you are obligated to accept or make.

I am only echoing the kind of principle promoted by WHO, because I think that the advice that I wish to share – based on current anti-viral research – is best framed that way. If a person at least manages to eat or drink five portions of food containing any of the anti-viral ingredients in this book, then they will be more likely (as opposed to doing nothing at all) to have a greater degree of protection against viruses and viral illnesses. The question of what could constitute a portion of each anti-viral ingredient, is one we will consider during the next section, along with some practical advice on incorporating the anti-viral ingredients into one's daily diet. It is my belief that the simple 'Anti-Viral 5-a-Day' principle offers the easiest way to get started with eating in an anti-viral way.

14. <u>CHOOSING DAILY MENUS</u>

THERE ARE THREE QUESTIONS which I would like to go some way towards answering in the current section. *Firstly*, how is one meant to think of portions - or servings - of the anti-viral ingredients? *Secondly*, in what general ways can one succeed in integrating these elements into one's own daily diet? And *lastly* - though I will not be providing a cookbook of recipes here - what more specific suggestions can be given concerning the meals and drinks we consume throughout the day?

To answer the last question, I have included a series of panels over the remainder of this chapter. These will hopefully give you some practical ideas about how - in quite a general sense - you can make the anti-viral ingredients a part of your diet. We consider a few options for the different meals of the day - breakfast, lunch and dinner - as well as considering snacks and beverages. All these can be a successful way to intake anti-viral ingredients. I think those panels are self-explanatory though I will be making a number of key points about these different meals and modes of ingestion shortly.

Turning to the first question, therefore - as it is quite a pressing one - *What is one meant to think of as a portion of an anti-viral ingredient? Can some specific advice be given?*

Thankfully, in the case of almost half the ingredients - certainly the Vitamins, Minerals, other Nutrients and Fruit or Vegetable ingredients - the ability to give advice on what can constitute a serving or portion (I use these words interchangeably) is assisted by the '5-a-Day' advice that WHO gives about portions of Fruit and Vegetables. Recommended Daily Allowances (RDAs) that are known for specific chemical compounds - *e.g.* L-Carnitine, Boron or Vitamin E - are also useful.

Eating an apple or banana, or a regular portion of fresh salad onyour dinner-plate - in the same way that each would constitute one portion of your 5-a-Day in terms of WHO's guideline, if you eat a piece of fruit with Quercetin in it (like an apple), then you can consider yourself as having had one serving of that anti-viral ingredient. Of course, in the case of a fruit like grapes or an ingredient like haricot beans, an *average portion* should be calculated, and in the case of WHO such a serving averages out at 80g as they estimate 400g of fruit and vegetables as a daily minimum - giving weight to it.

As *excess* intake - even of vitamins and minerals - can be just as dangerous as deficiency, a portion of any nutrient, including micronutrients, cannot exceed the maximum allowable daily amount. But, in a general sense, when someone has eaten a regular portion of food that is *rich* in one of the anti-viral ingredients presented here, then they have had one of their 'Anti-Viral 5-a-Day' - for example, a piece of calve's liver in the case of L-Carnitine, a peanut-butter sandwich or bowl of cereal with apricots and almond in the case of Boron, or even just a packet of Sunflower Seeds for your Vitamin E.

BREAKFAST SUGGESTIONS

- Have a Fresh Fruit Juice (Citrus) or Smoothie [add some Spirulina in there if you want to]

- Eat Cereals enriched with Vitamins & Minerals [focusing on the **AVD** Vitamins & Minerals]

- Add Fresh Fruit & Manuka Honey to your Cereal

- Try Echinacea or Green Tea instead of Coffee

- Enjoy Eggs, Salmon or Liver as part of a Hot Breakfast - maybe with Maitake & Sauerkraut

- Have Toast with Elderberry Jam or Manuka Honey & Fresh Fruit Pieces - for example, Apple, Banana

Without labouring the point, but just so as to make the advice as clear as possible, in the case of fruits and vegetables that are rich in any of the anti-viral ingredients, what would constitute a portion of that food under WHO's guidelines - is the same as what would constitute a portion of the anti-viral ingredient, in this diet. An average portion of any other food (meat, fish, protein substitutes, cereals *etc.*) can be estimated at 80g - just as in the case of fruit and vegetables - and if that food is rich in one of the anti-viral ingredients, then that would constitute a single portion of that ingredient.

As for those nutrients with specified Recommended Daily Intake (or Recommended Daily Allowance), that amount can be taken to be equivalent to one portion of the anti-viral ingredient in question. In all instances, the amount of the micronutrient being taken - whether in the form of food, or supplements - must never exceed the *maximum allowed* daily amount as there is a danger of toxicity or other negative outcomes.

MEAL SUGGESTIONS

- Have King-Prawns in a Ginger Marinade Stir-Fry & Black Rice [with **AVD** Herbs & Spices]

- Eat a Reishi Mushroom Omelette with Fried Potatoes seasoned with Oregano & Sage

- Try Fried Blue Fin Tuna & Grilled Artichokes with a Cream Cheese or Garlic Aoili Dip

- Have Grilled Sea Bass, Mashed Sweet Potato and a Dandelion Salad with Lemon & Olive Oil

- Eat Filet Mignon Steak in a Garlic & Rosemary Rub with Buckwheat Groats & Fermented Beets

---

However, there are other ingredients of the anti-viral diet about which some people may be struggling to understand what is being recommended as one portion. I think that there is more obscurity, for example, in relation to the ingredients that have been listed as herbs, spices, plants or flowers. They account for almost one third of the dietary elements overall, so there is a need to know how to calculate what *one portion* of each of them is, at least in an approximate way.

The ingredients set apart in the section 'Herbs & Spices' are suitable for a different purpose than 'Plants and Flowers', and that is the main reason why they have been placed in these separate sections. Herbs and spices are the kind of ingredients that are used within a sauce for flavour; as condiments for meat, fish and other proteins; or in the seasoning of a salad. The amount of that herb or spice in the average portion of the food served - and I would not recommend eating over-size portions unless your body is *in need* of extra - may

SNACK SUGGESTIONS

- Have One or more Pieces of Fruit or Fruit Salad [vary it so as to gain from different **AVD** ingredients]

- Eat a Cereal Bar rich in Nuts and Dried Fruits [Variety is best; with Brazil Nuts for Selenium]

- Have Fresh Fruit Juice or Smoothie (No Squash)

- Snack on Sesame, Pumpkin or Sunflower Seeds

- Have a Pizza Slice with assorted Anti-Viral Herbs

- Eat a Fortified Cereal any time - with Fruit & Nuts

- Try Celery or Carrot with an Olive Oil Mayo Dip

be considered to be one portion of that anti-viral ingredient in this diet. Herbs and spices are generally potent compounds, so there is no need to have any of them in a large quantity – although the amounts that may be effective are certainly of a greater size than the micro-portions of some nutrients (like vitamins and minerals) that are required by the human body.

As for the plants and flowers – in the 6th section of ingredients, these are generally ideal for preparing as beverages – and there are two general pieces of advice that I think may be of some guidance. In terms of using the leaves or petals of a plant so to make an infusion, the average contents of a tea-bag (a usual herbal/tea bag) are a sensible measure of what constitutes one portion of the anti-viral ingredient. If you have a tea-bag of pure Echinacea, for example, then one mug with hot water added will be the equivalent of a portion of that anti-viral element. However, in the case of some of other ingredients which take the form of roots, twigs or bark,

---

BEVERAGE SUGGESTIONS

- Try a Chilled Peppermint Tea with Lemon [or Orange or Lime, and leave the slice in there]

- Have a Fresh Fruit Juice – Apple or Orange [add a dash of Cider Vinegar for Fermented Element]

- Make a Licorice Infusion & add Manuka Honey

- Have a Vegetable Smoothie & be Adventurous [use Aspagarus, Celery, Carrots, even Broccoli]

- Drink Kefir or a Yoghurt Drink [both Fermented]

- Brew a Hibiscus Tea and add Sliced Ginger

- Sip a Glass of Red Wine (Madiran/Shiraz)

MY ANTI-VIRAL 5-A-DAY

1.

2.

3.

4.

5.

a beverage is more effectively prepared by bringing water to boil with the ingredient in the pot from the start, being left to simmer for usually something like 15 minutes. In the case of burdock root, for example, cat's claw, astragalus or liquorice, this is a method of preparation that has shown greater efficiency in drawing bioactive, medicinal compounds into the water. In the case of these types of ingredient, 1-2 teaspoons per mug/person will usually serve well as a general rule, and one mug of the beverage will once again be roughly equivalent to one portion of the anti-viral ingredient in this diet.

Hopefully, the general advice above, regarding average servings of the anti-viral ingredients, will have given you a better idea of how to approach **AVD** in terms of managing *5-a-Day*. Hopefully also, the four panels on the preceding pages will have given you an idea of what to do with breakfast, meals, snacks and beverages. Now note down your initial Anti-Viral 5-a-Day in the box above - *and make a start.*

15. <u>COMMENCING A DIET</u>

"STARTING IS HALF THE TASK" is one of the truest proverbs I have ever come across. That is why, if you have not yet done so - but *are* interested in giving this diet a try - I would highly recommend that you return to the previous page and fill in an initial 'Anti-Viral Five-a-Day' for yourself to consider taking. If you have filled in your top twenty anti-viral ingredients on pages 178-179 before, then you might want to choose five items out of that list to try out on your first **AVD** day. The thing is that once you have written down a list, it becomes far easier for you to make a start. So if this is something that you do really want to try out, jot down your first 5 starting ingredients in the box on the previous page or on any piece of notepaper. Ideally return to this chapter once you have done that.

You will find yourself in a better position to consider what you think about this diet once you have eaten your first portion, especially after your first day. The point is, there is no no need to make starting a diet into a big thing. You eat food every day anyway, and all of the foods in this book are non-toxic and safe. But remember, as stressed in Section 12, certain safety precautions have to be taken regarding this diet.

If however, you have not made your mind up on this proposal of an anti-viral diet, and wish to read **Parts 1** and **2**, - perhaps even review some of the research dossiers online *before* making a decision - then that is no problem at all. Deciding what to eat on an everyday basis is an important decision and there is no need to make your choice in an instant.

Nonetheless, I am aware that there will be some who have come to this diet - particularly since it has been updated with evidence regarding COVID-19 - in order to find a dietary treatment option for that illness. I will not deny that this diet *may be of help*, but **no promises or guarantees** are being made that **AVD** will successfully treat COVID-19 or any other condition. There is a *degree of probability* that eating at least five anti-viral ingredients a day may increase the effectiveness of your immune system and may offer you more viral protection. However, as the way in which a person's body responds to medication and food - and other factors - is not something that can ever be predicted, this diet is only presented as a general approach and not as any type of targeted treatment.

The *Anti-Viral Five-a-Day* is only presented as a principle for making sure you get a minimum effective amount of anti-viral ingredients. However, you can certainly eat more of them, as long as you never exceed maximum RDIs. As far as the positive effect of eating more fruit and vegetables per day is concerned, Imperial College London published results from a study undertaken by a group of ten researchers, in the International Journal of Epidemiology (2017), that confirmed:

"*for coronary heart disease, stroke, cardiovascular disease and all-cause mortality the lowest risk was observed at 800 g/day (10 servings/day), a level of intake that is double the five servings per day (400 g/day) currently recommended by the World Cancer Research Fund, the WHO, and in England.*"

There is no reason to believe that having more anti-viral ingredients per day will not also be *more* rather than *less* beneficial, potentially increasing one's level of viral protection and general immunity. What must be severely warned against is adopting any kind of 'Crash Diet' - where you expose yourself to excess quantities in a short time. *That may cause harm.*

The one thing that I am sure about though, is that there is no way in which anyone will be able to find out if an anti-viral diet - containing potential natural anti-virals and immuno-enhancing elements - is effective, if they don't give it a try. Only if you try something out, can you see if it works in reality.

16. REVIEWING AVD

THE ONLY WAY THAT YOU WILL ever know if this diet is beneficial for *you*, is if it is successful in protecting you from illness. There are a few possible ways in which you could become aware of its effectiveness. If, after a considerable period of time following this diet, you have not fallen ill from colds, influenzas or other viral illnesses as often as you did before, you might take that as personal evidence of its working. Or you could just chalk it down to good luck, not getting ill during that time. On the other hand, if you are suffering from an illness right now, and after following this diet for only a few days you recover successfully, it could be that you believe it is the reason that you have got better. Of course, there is no excluding other factors being responsible for your recovery, but the longer the period of time goes by in which you do not fall ill, the more likely you will give some credence to the possibility that these natural ingredients may offer viral protection.

In any case, I highly recommend that anyone who follows this diet should review how it is working for them regularly. If you are unsure that you are eating enough of the ingredients, in the right quantity, or from enough different groups, then take some time out to consider what you are doing and reconsider the whole range of ingredients in **Part 2** of **AVD**. The one thing that will be advocated here - especially if you are returning to this book after trying this diet already and are reviewing choices – is that the human body needs the widest variety of beneficial ingredients in order to function at its best. If you are not already doing so, then choose a few ingredients from *each* of the sections of **Part 2**. It is probable that a wider variety of anti-viral compounds will have a greater effect.

One thing that *will be guaranteed here*, is that the Anti-Viral Diet in this publication will be reviewed and updated on a continual basis. The online supplementary research dossiers

194

are not a static resource – the evidence in support of the anti-viral and immuno-supportive aspects of the **AVD** ingredients is being reconsidered and added to as the results of further research, experimentation and trials emerge. As was emphasized at numerous points during this publication, **AVD** is not a completed diet but one which will continue to develop and transform as we see how natural chemical agents demonstrate their potential in clinical trials over the coming years.

I am not going to try and respond – in advance – to all of the possible negative criticisms and invective which will be launched against **AVD** – there is just no point. The Anti-Viral Diet is a proposition, not a prescription. It is not claimed as a 'true diet' but as a potentially therapeutic one whose effectiveness may be better evidenced in time, as the results of further investigations come in. For those who wish to follow how scientific research is impacting this diet, please log onto the site www.theantiviraldiet.com, where the links to current research on all aspects of this diet are being regularly updated.

From my own perspective, this book has been one that I did not so much choose to write, but one that I felt obliged to write. Personally, I found myself convinced by the research that had been taking place over the past century – and above all over the last fifty years – that an anti-viral diet is a viable project, one that should continue to be pursued as an ideal until a scientifically proven anti-viral diet ultimately exists.

What I hold as an ideal for such a diet, is that it should offer maximum protection from viruses (and viral illnesses) by specifying the most effective ingredients at inhibiting viruses and optimizing the immune system's response to all threats. That such a diet is not yet proven, is a fact. But from my own personal perspective, I already believe in the effectiveness of a diet such as I have shared with you here – because just a handful of the ingredients that I have presented to you in this book have protected me from illness for many years. It is my sincere hope that **AVD** may prove to be just as beneficial to you.

PART 3 CREATING YOUR DIET
KEY POINTS

1. *The First Stage in Creating Your Own Anti-Viral Diet comes with Selecting a Range of Anti-Viral Ingredients from **Part 2** of this Diet Program*

2. *Choice of Ingredients needs to be made with Several Safety Precautions in mind - for example, taking into account Allergies, Illnesses and Medications*

3. *The Principle of an 'Anti-Viral 5-a-Day' is proposed so as to help Get You Started with an Anti-Viral Diet in the Simplest Way Possible - with 5 Ingredients*

4. *Calculating the Portions or Servings of Anti-Viral Ingredients can be done in a Similar Way to the Calculation of a Fruit-&-Vegetable '5-a-Day'*

5. *Increasing your '5-a-Day' to an 'Anti-Viral 10-a-Day' will likely Increase Your Degree of Protection against Viruses*

6. *Reviewing the Effect of Your Anti-Viral Diet on Your Health is Highly Advisable - Adjust Your Diet According to Results*

7. *The Anti-Viral Diet is being Continuously Reviewed in line with Scientific Evidence*

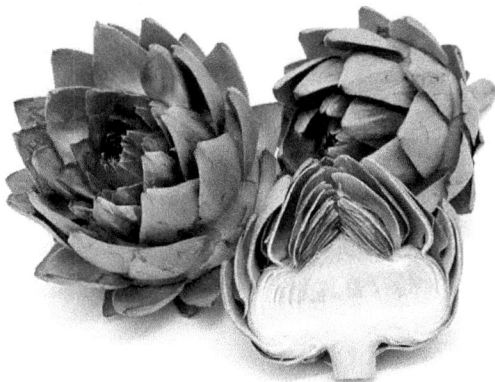

"Functional foods' prevention of non-communicable disease can be translated into protecting against respiratory viral infections and COVID-19. Functional foods and nutraceuticals within popular diets contain immune-boosting nutraceuticals, polyphenols, terpenoids, flavonoids, alkaloids, sterols, pigments, unsaturated fatty-acids, micronutrient vitamins and minerals, including vitamin A, B6, B12, C, D, E, and folate, and trace elements, including zinc, iron, selenium, magnesium, and copper. Foods with antiviral properties include fruits, vegetables, fermented foods and probiotics, olive oil, fish, nuts and seeds, herbs, roots, fungi, amino acids, peptides, and cyclotides."

DR. AHMAD ALKHATIB

APPENDIX

RESEARCH REFERENCES

Please note that this is only a Select Bibliography of a small number of papers that have been referred to when deciding upon the inclusion of the 52 Ingredients in **Part 2** of **AVD**. More extensive bibliographies are available by clicking on the links in each section.

1 - *Enhancing Immunity in Viral Infections, with Special Emphasis on COVID-19: A Review* - Ranil Jayawardena, Piumika Sooriyaarachchi, Michail Chourdakis, Chandima Jeewandara & Priyanga Ranasinghe - **Diabetology & Metabolic Syndrome** (Jul-Aug. 2020).

2 - *Potential Interventions for Novel Coronavirus in China: A Systematic Review* - Lei Zhang & Yunhui Liu - **Journal of Medical Virology** (13 Feb. 2020).

3 - *COVID-19: is there a Role for Immunonutrition, particularly in the Over 65s?* - Emma Derbyshire & Joanne Delange - **BMJ Nutrition, Prevention & Health** (4 May 2020).

4 - *Quercetin and Vitamin C: An Experimental, Synergistic Therapy for the Prevention and Treatment of SARS-CoV-2 Related Disease (COVID-19)* - Ruben Manuel Luciano Colunga Biancatelli, Max Berrill, John D. Catravas & Paul E. Marik - **Frontiers in Immunology** (19 Jun. 2020).

5 - *Vitamin D Supplementation: A Potential Approach for Coronavirus/COVID-19 Therapeutics?* - John F. Arboleda & Silvio Urcuqui-Inchima - **Frontiers in Immunology** (23 Jun. 2020).

6 - *Effects of Micronutrients or Conditional Amino Acids on COVID-19-Related Outcomes: An Evidence Analysis Center Scoping Review* - Mary Rozga, Feon W. Cheng, Lisa Moloney & Deepa Handu - **Journal of the Academy of Nutrition and Dietetics** (2020).

7 - Potential Role of Zinc Supplementation in Prophylaxis and Treatment of COVID-19 - Amit Kumar, Yuichi Kubota, Mikhail Chernov & Hidetoshi Kasuya - **Medical Hypotheses** (25 May 2020).

8 - The Potential Impact of Zinc Supplementation on COVID-19 Pathogenesis - Inga Wessels, Benjamin Rolles & Lothar Rink - **Frontiers in Immunology** (10 Jul. 2020).

9 - Serum Iron Level as a Potential Predictor of Coronavirus Disease 2019 Severity and Mortality: A Retrospective Study - Kang Zhao, Jucun Huang, Dan Dai, Yuwei Feng, Liming Liu & Shuke Nie - **Open Forum Infectious Diseases** (21 Jun. 2020).

10 - Depriving Iron Supply to the Virus Represents a Promising Adjuvant Therapeutic Against Viral Survival - Wei Liu, Shu-ping Zhang, Sergei Nekhai & Sijin Liu - **Current Clinical Microbiology Reports** (20 Apr. 2020).

11 - Combating COVID-19 and Building Immune Resilience: A Potential Role for Magnesium Nutrition? - Taylor C. Wallace - **Journal of the American College of Nutrition** (13 May 2020).

12 - Magnesium Deficiency and COVID- 19 - What are the Links? - Oliver Micke, Jürgen Vormann & Klaus Kisters - **Trace Elements and Electrolytes**; **Munich** (2020).

13 - Innate Immune Cells Speak Manganese - Hajo Haase - **Immunity** (17 Apr. 2018).

14 - Nutritional Immunity Beyond Iron: A Role for Manganese and Zinc - Thomas E. Kehl-Fie & Eric P. Skaar - **Current Opinion in Chemical Biology** (Apr. 2010).

15 - Association between Regional Selenium Status and Reported Outcome of COVID-19 Cases in China - Jinsong

Zhang, Ethan Will Taylor, Kate Bennett, Ramy Saad & Margaret P. Rayman - **The American Journal of Clinical Nutrition** (8 Apr. 2020).

16 - *Selenium and Viral Infection: Are there Lessons for COVID-19?* - G. Bermano, C. Méplan, D.K. Mercer & J.E. Hesketh - **British Journal of Nutrition** (6 Aug. 2020).

17 - *Boron in Human Health: Evidence for Dietary Recommendations and Public Policies* - S. Meacham, S. Karakas, A. Wallace & F. Altun - **The Open Mineral Processsing Journal** (2010).

18 - *Growing Evidence for Human Health Benefits of Boron* - Forrest H. Nielsen & Susan L. Meacham - **Journal of Evidence-Based Complementary & Alternative Medicine** (2011).

19 - *Effects of Copper Deficiency on the Immune System* - Joseph R. Prohaska & Omelan A. Lukasewycz - from **Antioxidant Nutrients and Immune Functions** (1990).

20 - *The Potential Beneficial Effect of EPA and DHA Supplementation Managing Cytokine Storm in Coronavirus Disease* - Zoltán Szabó, Tamás Marosvölgyi, Éva Szabó, Péter Bai, Mária Figler & Zsófia Verzár - **Frontiers in Physiology** (19 Jun. 2020).

21 - *Potential Benefits and Risks of Omega-3 Fatty Acids Supplementation to Patients with COVID-19* - Marcelo M. Rogero, Matheus de C. Leão, Tamires M. Santana, Mariana V. de M.B. Pimentel, Giovanna C.G. Carlini, Tayse F.F. da Silveira, Renata C. Gonçalves & Inar A. Castro - **Free Radicals in Biological Medicine** (10 Jul. 2020).

22 - *Alpha-Lipoic Acid may protect Patients with Diabetes against COVID-19 Infection* - Erkan Cure & Medine Cumhur Cure - **Medical Hypotheses** (Oct. 2020).

23 - *Carotenoid Action on the Immune Response* - Boon P. Chew & Jean Soon Park - **The Journal of Nutrition** (Jan. 2004).

24 - *β-Carotene and the Immune Response* - Adrianne Bendich - **Proceedings of the Nutrition Society** (Aug. 1991).

25 - *β-Glucan Extracts from the same Edible Shiitake Mushroom Lentinus Edodes produce Differential In-Vitro Immunomodulatory and Pulmonary Cytoprotective Effects* — Implications for Coronavirus Disease (COVID-19) Immunotherapies - Emma J. Murphy, Claire Masterson, Emanuele Rezoagli, Daniel O'Toole, Ian Major, Gary D. Stack, Mark Lynch, John G. Laffey & Neil J. Rowan - **Science of the Total Environment** (25 Aug. 2020).

26 - *The Antiviral, Anti-Inflammatory Effects of Natural Medicinal Herbs and Mushrooms and SARS-CoV-2 Infection* - Fanila Shahzad, Diana Anderson & Mojgan Najafzadeh - **nutrients** (25 Aug. 2020).

27 - *L-Carnitine can Extinguish the COVID19 Fire: A Review on Molecular Aspects* - Mohammad Fakhrolmobasheri, Hossein Khanahmad, Mohammad Javad Kahlani, Amir Abbas Shiravi, Seyedeh Ghazal Shahrokh & Mehrdad Zeinalian - **zenodo** (4 Apr. 2020).

28 - *Carnitine and Derivatives in Experimental Infections* - Nicola M. Kouttab, Linda L. Gallo, Dwayne Ford, Chris Galanos & Michael Chirigos - from **Carnitine Today** (1997).

29 - *Effect of Quercetin on Prophylaxis and Treatment of COVID-19* - Kanuni Sultan Suleyman Training and Research Hospital - **ClinicalTrials.gov** (May 6, 2020).

30 - *The Effect of Quercetin on the Prevention or Treatment of COVID-19 and Other Respiratory Tract Infections in Humans: A Rapid Review* - Monique Aucoin, Kieran Cooley, Paul

Richard Saunders, Valentina Cardozo, Daniella Remy, Holger Cramer, Carlos Neyre Abad & Nicole Hannan - **Advances in Integrative Medicine** (30 Jul. 2020).

31 - *Could the Inhibition of Endo-Lysosomal Two-Pore Channels (TPCs) by the Natural Flavonoid Naringenin represent an Option to Fight SARS-CoV-2 Infection?* - Antonio Filippini, Antonella D'Amore, Fioretta Palombi & Armando Carpaneto - **Frontiers in Microbiology** (30 Apr. 2020).

32 - *Naringenin, a Flavanone with Antiviral and Anti-Inflammatory Effects: A Promising Treatment Strategy against COVID-19* - Helda Tutunchi, Fatemeh Naeini, Alireza Ostadrahimi & Mohammad Javad Hosseinzadeh-Attar - **Phytotherapy Research** (2 Jul. 2020).

33 - *Is Hesperidin Essential for Prophylaxis and Treatment of COVID-19 Infection?* - Yusuf A. Haggag, Nahla E. El-Ashmawy & Kamal M. Okashac - **Medical Hypotheses** (6 Jun. 2020).

34 - *Hesperidin and SARS-CoV-2: New Light on the Healthy Functions of Citrus Fruit* - Paolo Bellavite & Alberto Donzelli - **PrePrints** (28 Jun. 2020).

35 - *Targeting SARS-CoV-2 Spike Protein of COVID-19 with Naturally Occurring Phytochemicals: An In Silico Study for Drug Development* - Jitendra Subhash Rane, Aroni Chatterjee, Abhijeet Kumar & Shashikant Ray - **chemRxiv** (8 Apr. 2020).

36 - *The Therapeutic Potential of Apigenin* - Bahare Salehi, Alessandro Venditti, Mehdi Sharifi-Rad, Dorota Kręgiel, Javad Sharifi-Rad, Alessandra Durazzo, Massimo Lucarini, Antonello Santini, Eliana B. Souto, Ettore Novellino, Hubert Antolak, Elena Azzini, William N. Setzer & Natália Martins - **International Journal of Molecular Science** (15 Mar. 2019).

37 - *In Silico Exploration of Repurposing and Optimizing Traditional Chinese Medicine Rutin for Possibly Inhibiting SARS-CoV-2's Main Protease* - Tien Huynh, Haoran Wang, Wendy Cornell & Binquan Luan - **ChemRxiv** (11 May 2020).

38 - *Possible SARS-Coronavirus 2 Inhibitor revealed by Simulated Molecular Docking to Viral Main Protease and Host toll-like Receptor* - Xiaopeng Hu, Xin Cai, Xun Song, Chenyang Li, Jia Zhao, Wenli Luo, Qian Zhang, Ivo Otte Ekumi & Zhendan He - **Future Virology** (12 Jun. 2020).

39 - *Evaluation of Green Tea Polyphenols as Novel Corona Virus (SARS CoV-2) Main Protease (Mpro) Inhibitors – An In Silico Docking and Molecular Dynamics Simulation Study* - Rajesh Ghosh, Ayon Chakraborty, Ashis Biswas & Snehasis Chowdhuri - **Journal of Biomolecular Structure and Dynamics** (22 Jun 2020).

40 - *Antiviral Activity of Green Tea and Black Tea Polyphenols in Prophylaxis and Treatment of COVID-19: A Review* - Susmit Mhatre, Tishya Srivastava, Shivraj Naik & Vandana Patravale - **Phytomedicine** (17 Jul. 2020).

41 - *Green Tea and Spirulina Extracts inhibit SARS, MERS, and SARS-2 Spike Pseudotyped Virus Entry In Vitro* - Jeswin Joseph, Karthika T., Ariya Ajay, V.R. Akshay Das & Stalin Raj - **bioRxiv** (23 Jun. 2020).

42 - *Investigation into SARS-CoV-2 Resistance of Compounds in Garlic Essential Oil* - Bui Thi Phuong Thuy, Tran Thi Ai My, Nguyen Thi Thanh Hai, Le Trung Hieu, Tran Thai Hoa, Huynh Thi Phuong Loan, Nguyen Thanh Triet, Tran Thi Van Anh, Phan Tu Quy, Pham Van Tat, Nguyen Van Hue, Duong Tuan Quang, Nguyen Tien Trung, Vo Thanh Tung, Lam K. Huynh & Nguyen Thi Ai Nhung - **ACS Omega** (31 Mar. 2020).

43 - *Discovery of Allicin as a Putative Inhibitor of the Main*

Protease of SARS-CoV-2 by Molecular Docking – Bijun Cheng & Tianjiao Li – **Biotechniques** (27 May 2020).

44 – *The Effects of Allium Sativum on Immunity within the Scope of COVID-19 Infection* – Mustafa Metin Donma & Orkide Donma – **Medical Hypotheses** (2 Jun. 2020).

45 – *Revealing the Potency of Citrus and Galangal Constituents to halt SARS-CoV-2 Infection* – Rohmad Yudi Utomo, Muthi' Ikawati & Edy Meiyanto – **PrePrints** [Basel] (12 Mar. 2020).

46 – *Natural Product Compounds in Alpinia Officinarum and Ginger are Potent SARS-CoV-2 Papain-like Protease Inhibitors* – Dibakar Goswami, Mukesh Kumar, Sunil K. Ghosh & Amit Das – **ChemRxiv** (5 Apr. 2020).

47 – *Virtual Screening of Curcumin and Its Analogs Against the Spike Surface Glycoprotein of SARS-CoV-2 and SARS-CoV* – Ashish Patel, Malathi Rajendran, Suresh B. Pakala, Ashish Shah, Harnisha Patel & Prashanthi Karyala – **ChemRxiv** (26 Apr. 2020).

48 – *Curcumin: a Wonder Drug as a Preventive Measure for COVID-19 Management* – Yamuna Manoharan, Vikram Haridas, K.C. Vasanthakumar, Sundaram Muthu, Fathima F. Thavoorullah & Praveenkumar Shetty – **Indian Journal of Clinical Biochemistry** (17 Jun. 2020).

49 – *Phytochemical 6-Gingerol - A Promising Drug of Choice for COVID-19* – Thirumalaisamy Rathinavel, Murugan Palanisamy, Palanisamy Srinivasan, Arjunan Subramanian & Selvankumar Thangaswamy – **ResearchGate** (May 2020).

50 – *Activity of Phytochemical Constituents of Black Pepper, Ginger, and Garlic against Coronavirus (COVID-19): An In Silico Approach* – Kalirajan Rajagopal, Gowramma Byran,

Srikanth Jupudi & R. Vadivelan - **International Journal of Health and Allied Sciences** (4 Jun. 2020).

51 - *Natural Product Compounds in Alpinia Officinarum and Ginger are Potent SARS-CoV-2 Papain-like Protease Inhibitors* - Dibakar Goswami, Mukesh Kumar, Sunil K. Ghosh & Amit Das - **ChemRxiv** (5 Apr. 2020).

52 - In Silico Investigation of Spice Molecules as Potent Inhibitor of SARS-CoV-2 - Janmejaya Rout, Bikash Chandra Swain & Umakanta Tripathy - **Indian Institute of Technology, Dhanbad** (2020).

53 - *Structure-based Drug Designing for Potential Antiviral Activity of Selected Natural Products from Ayurveda against SARS-CoV-2 Spike Glycoprotein and its Cellular Receptor* - Vimal K. Maurya, Swatantra Kumar, Anil K. Prasad, Madan L.B. Bhatt & Shailendra K. Saxena - **VirusDisease** (24 May 2020).

54 - *Investigation of Rosemary Herbal Extracts (Rosmarinus Officinalis) and their Potential Effects on Immunity* - Hiwa M. Ahmed & Muhammed Babakir Mina - **Phytotherapy Research** (22 Feb. 2020).

55 - *Preliminary Identification of Hamamelitannin and Rosmarinic Acid as COVID-19 Inhibitors Based on Molecular Docking* - Kaushik Sarkar & Rajesh Das - **Letters in Drug Design & Discovery** (Aug. 2020).

56 - *Antiviral Properties of Supercritical CO2 Extracts from Oregano and Sage* - S. Santoyo, L. Jaime, M.R. García-Risco, A. Ruiz-Rodríguez & G. Reglero - **International Journal of Food Properties** (14 Jan 2014).

57 - *Evaluation of Antiviral Activity of Fractionated Extracts of Sage Salvia Officinalis L. (Lamiaceae)* - Dragana Šmidling,

Dragana Mitić-Ćulafić, Branka Vuković-Gačić & Draga Simić - **Archives of Biological Sciences** (Jan. 2008).

58 - *Effective Antiviral Activity of Essential Oils and their Characteristics Terpenes against Coronaviruses: An Update* - Mohamed Nadjib Boukhatem - **ResearchGate** (Mar. 2020).

59 - *Aqueous Extracts from Peppermint, Sage and Lemon Balm Leaves display Potent Anti-HIV-1 Activity by increasing the Virion Density* - Silvia Geuenich, Christine Goffinet, Stephanie Venzke, Silke Nolkemper, Ingo Baumann, Peter Plinkert, Jürgen Reichling & Oliver T. Keppler - **Retrovirology** (20 Mar. 2008).

60 - *Antiviral Activities of Extracts and Selected Pure Constituents of Ocimum Basilicum* - Chiang L.C., Ng L.T., Cheng P.W., Chiang W. & Lin C.C. - **Clinical and Experimental Pharmacology and Physiology** (Oct. 2005).

61 - *Evaluation of Antiviral Activity of Ocimum Sanctum and Acacia Arabica Leaves Extracts against H9N2 Virus using Embryonated Chicken Egg Model* - S.S. Ghoke, R. Sood , N. Kumar, A.K. Pateriya, S. Bhatia, A. Mishra, R. Dixit, V.K. Singh, D.N. Desai, D.D. Kulkarni, U. Dimri & V.P. Singh - **BMC Complementary and Alternative Medicine** (5 Jun. 2018).

62 - *Pharmacological Perspective: Glycyrrhizin may be an Efficacious Therapeutic Agent for COVID-19* - Pan Luo, Dong Liu & Juan Li - **International Journal of Antimicrobial Agents** (24 Apr. 2020).

63 - *Glycyrrhizin: An Alternative Drug for the Treatment of COVID-19 Infection and the Associated Respiratory Syndrome?* - Christian Bailly & Gérard Vergoten - **Pharmacology and Therapeutics** (24 Jun. 2020).

64 - *Shenhuang Granule in the Treatment of Severe Corona-virus Disease 2019 (COVID-19): Study Protocol for an Open-Label Randomized Controlled Clinical Trial* - Bangjiang Fang, Wen Zhang, Xinxin Wu, Tingrong Huang, Huacheng Li, You Zheng, Jinhua Che, Shuting Sun, Chao Jiang, Shuang Zhou & Jun Feng - **Trials** (24 Jun. 2020). [Panax Ginseng is one of 6 Ingredients of the Granule being tested in Trial.]

65 - *Antiviral, Embryo Toxic and Cytotoxic Activities of Astragalus Membranaceus Root Extracts* - Khan H.M., Raza S.M., Anjum A.A. & Ali M.A. - **Pakistan Journal of Pharmaceutical Sciences** (Jan. 2019).

66 - *Potential Source for HSV-1 Therapy by Acting on Virus or the Susceptibility of Host* - Wen Li, Xiao-Hua Wang, Zhuo Luo, Li-Fang Liu, Chang Yan, Chang-Yu Yan, Guo-Dong Chen, Hao Gao, Wen-Jun Duan, Hiroshi Kurihara, Yi-Fang Li & Rong-Rong He - **International Journal of Molecular Science** (20 Oct. 2018).

67 - *The Role of Andrographolide and its Derivative in COVID-19 associated Proteins and Immune System* - Yadu Nandan Dey, Pukar Khanal, B.M. Patil, Manish M. Wanjari, Bhavana Srivastava, Shailendra S. Gurav & Sudesh N. Gaidhani - **Immunology Infectious Diseases** (18 Jun. 2020).

68 - *Andrographolide as a Potential Inhibitor of SARS-CoV-2 Main Protease: An In Silico Approach* - Sukanth Kumar Enmozhi, Kavitha Raja, Irudhayasamy Sebastine & Jerrine Joseph - **Journal of Biomolecular Structure and Dynamics** (5 May 2020).

69 - *Investigating Potential Inhibitory Effect of Uncaria Tomentosa (Cat's Claw) against the Main Protease 3CLPro of SARS-CoV-2 by Molecular Modeling* - Andres F. Yepes-Pérez, Oscar Herrera-Calderon, José-Emilio Sánchez-Aparicio, Laura

Tiessler-Sala, Jean-Didier Maréchal & Wilson Cardona-G. - **PrePrints** (28 Jun. 2020).

70 - *Immunomodulating and Antiviral Activities of Uncaria Tomentosa on Human Monocytes infected with Dengue Virus-2* - Reis S.R., Valente L.M., Sampaio A.L., Siani A.C., Gandini M., Azeredo E.L., D'Avila L.A., Mazzei J.L., Henriques M. & Kubelka C.F. - **International Immunopharmacology** (26 Dec. 2007).

71 - *Anti-Influenza Virus Effect of Aqueous Extracts from Dandelion* - He W., Han H., Wang W. & Gao B. - **Virology Journal** (14 Dec. 2011).

72 - *Comparison of the Immunomodulatory Properties of Root and Leaves of Arctium Lappa (Burdock) In Vitro* - Hasan Namdar, Morteza Behnamfar, Maryam Nezafat Firizi & Sahar Saghayan - **Zahedan Journal of Research in Medical Sciences** (28 Oct. 2017).

73 - *Antiviral Activity of the Oseltamivir and Melissa Officinalis L. Essential Oil against Avian Influenza A Virus (H9N2)* - Gholamhosein Pourghanbari, Hasan Nili, Afagh Moattari, Ali Mohammadi & Aida Iraji - **Virusdisease** (21 May 2016).

74 - *The Effect of the Melissa Officinalis Extract on Immune Response in Mice* - Drozd J. & Anuszewska E. - **Acta Poloniae Pharmaceutica** (Nov-Dec. 2003).

75 - *In Vitro Antiviral Activity of Echinaforce®, an Echinacea Purpurea Preparation, against Common Cold Coronavirus 229E and Highly Pathogenic MERS-CoV and SARS-CoV* - Johanna Signer, Hulda R. Jonsdottir, Werner C. Albrich, Marc Strasser, Roland Züst, Sarah Ryter, Rahel Ackermann-Gäumann, Nicole Lenz, Denise Siegrist, Andreas Suter, Roland Schoop & Olivier B. Engler - **Research Square** (26 Feb./10 Mar./15 Aug. 2020).

76 - *Echinacea Purpurea to treat Novel Coronavirus (2019-nCoV)* - R. Anandan, Suseendran G., Noor Zaman & Sarfraz N. Brohi - **ResearchGate** (May 2020).

77 - *Can Hypericum Perforatum (SJW) prevent Cytokine Storm in COVID-19 Patients?* - Pellegrino Masiello, Michela Novelli, Pascale Beffy & Marta Menegazzi - **Phytotherapy Research** (5 Jun. 2020).

78 - *Naturally occurring Anthraquinones as Potential Inhibitors of SARS-CoV-2 Main Protease: A Molecular Docking Study* - Sourav Das & Atanu Singha Roy - **Department of Chemistry, National Institute of Technology Meghalaya** (3 May 2020).

79 - *Immunomodulation by Hibiscus Rosa-Sinensis: Effect on the Humoral and Cellular Immune Response of Mus Musculus* - Nidhi Mishra, Vijay Lakshmi Tandon & Rekha Gupta - **Pakistan Journal of Biological Sciences** (15 Mar. 2012).

80 - *Antiviral Activities of Hibiscus Sabdariffa L. Tea Extract Against Human Influenza A Virus Rely Largely on Acidic pH but Partially on a Low-pH-Independent Mechanism* - Yohei Takeda, Yuko Okuyama, Hiroto Nakano, Yasunori Yaoita, Koich Machida, Haruko Ogawa & Kunitoshi Imai - **Food and Environmental Virology** (16 Oct. 2019).

81 - *Potential Contribution of Beneficial Microbes to face the COVID-19 Pandemic* - Adriane E.C. Antunes, Gabriel Vinderola, Douglas Xavier-Santos & Katia Sivieric - **Food Research International** (24 Jul. 2020).

82 - *Cabbage and Fermented Vegetables: From Death Rate Heterogeneity in Countries to Candidates for Mitigation Strategies of Severe COVID-19* - Jean Bousquet, Josep M. Anto, Wienczyslawa Czarlewski, Tari Haahtela, Susana C. Fonseca, Guido Iaccarino, Hubert Blain, Alain Vidal, Aziz

Sheikh, Cezmi A. Akdis & Torsten Zuberbier - **Allergy** (6 Aug. 2020).

83 - *In Silico Approach of Some Selected Honey Constituents as SARS-CoV-2 Main Protease (COVID-19) Inhibitors* - Heba E. Hashem - **Eurasian Journal of Medicine and Oncology** (5 May 2020).

84 - *Prospects of Honey in Fighting against COVID-19: Pharmacological Insights and Therapeutic Promises* - Khandkar Shaharina Hossain, Md. Golzar Hossain, Akhi Moni & Md. Mahbubur Rahman - **ResearchGate** (Jun. 2020).

85 - *Therapeutic and Nutritional Potential of Spirulina in Combating COVID-19 Infection* - Sunita D. Singh, Vinay Dwivedi, Debanjan Sanyal & Santanu Dasgupta - **Nutraceuticals from Microalgae** (May 2020).

86 - *Algae: A Potential Source to Prevent and Cure the Novel Coronavirus - A Review* - Elaya Perumal Ulagalanthaperumal & Sundararaj R. - **ResearchGate** (24 Apr. 2020).

87 - *Potential Inhibitor of COVID-19 Main Protease (Mpro) from Several Medicinal Plant Compounds by Molecular Docking Study* - Siti Khaerunnisa, Hendra Kurniawan, Rizki Awaluddin, Suhartati Suhartati & Soetjipto Soetjipto - **Pre-Prints** (13 Mar. 2020).

88 - *Antiviral Effects of Olea Europaea Leaves Extract and Interferon-beta on Gene Expression of Newcastle Disease Virus* - Rajaa Hindi Salih, Shony Mechail Odisho, Ahmed Majeed Al-Shammari, Orooba & Mohammed Saeed Ibrahim - **Advances in Animal and Veterinary Science** (15 Oct. 2015).

89 - *Natural Bioactive Compounds from Fungi as Potential Candidates for Protease Inhibitors and Immunomodulators to Apply for Coronaviruses* - Nakarin Suwannarach, Jaturong

Kumla, Kanaporn Sujarit, Thanawat Pattananandecha, Chalermpong Saenjum & Saisamorn Lumyong - **Molecules** (14 Apr. 2020).

90 - *Maitake Mushrooms (Grifola Frondosa) enhances Antibody Production in Response to Influenza Vaccination in Healthy Adult Volunteers concurrent with Alleviation of Common Cold Symptoms* - Jun Nishihira, Mayumi Sato, Aiko Tanaka, Masatoshi Okamatsu, Tomonori Azuma, Naonobu Tsutsumi & Shozo Yoneyama - **Functional Foods in Health & Disease** (2017).

91 - *Can Activation of NRF2 Be a Strategy against COVID-19?* - Antonio Cuadrado, Marta Pajares, Cristina Benito, Gina Manda, Ana I. Rojo & Albena T. Dinkova-Kostova - **Trends in Pharmacological Sciences** (14 Jul. 2020).

92 - *Antiviral Potential of Mushrooms in the Light of their Biological Active Compounds* - Waill A. Elkhateeb, Ghoson M. Daba, Elmahdy M. Elmahdy, Paul W. Thomas, Ting-Chi Wen & Mohamed N.F. Shaheen - **ARC Journal of Pharmaceutical Sciences** (2019).

93 - *Stilbene-based Natural Compounds as Promising Drug Candidates against COVID-19* - Wahedi H.M., Ahmad S. & Abbasi S.W. - **Journal of Biomolecular Structure and Dynamics** (12 May 2020).

94 - *Indomethacin and Resveratrol as Potential Treatment Adjuncts for SARS-CoV-2/COVID-19* - Mark A. Marinella - **International Journal of Clinical Practice** (15 May 2020).

95 - *Elderberry is Anti-Bacterial, Anti-Viral and Modulates the Immune System: Anti-Bacterial, Anti-Viral and Immunomodulatory Non-Clinical (In-Vitro) Effects of Elderberry Fruit and Flowers (Sambucus Nigra): A Systematic Review* - Julia Wermig-Morgan - **Doctoral Thesis, Oxford University** (Feb. 2020).

96 - *The Effects of Sambucus Nigra Berry on Acute Respiratory Viral infections: A Rapid Review of Clinical Studies* - Joanna Harnett, Kerrie Oakes, Jenny Carè, M. Leach, D. Brown, Holger Cramer, Tobey-Ann Pinder, A. Steel & D. Anheyer - **Advances in Integrative Medicine** (2020).

97 - *Geranium and Lemon Essential Oils and Their Active Compounds Downregulate Angiotensin-Converting Enzyme 2 (ACE2), a SARS-CoV-2 Spike Receptor-Binding Domain, in Epithelial Cells* - K.J. Senthil Kumar, M. Gokila Vani, Chung-Shuan Wang, Chia-Chi Chen, Yu-Chien Chen, Li-Ping Lu, Ching-Hsiang Huang, Chien-Sing Lai & Sheng-Yang Wang - **Plants** (Jun. 2020).

98 - *Immunomodulatory Activity of Naturally Occurring Monoterpenes Carvone, Limonene, and Perillic Acid* - T.J. Raphael & G. Kuttan - **Immunopharmacology and Immunotoxicology** (28 Apr. 2003).

99 - *Evaluation of Immunomodulatory Activity of Transanethole and Estragole, and Protective Effect against Cyclophosphamide-induced Suppression of Immunity in Swiss Albino Mice* - L.A.M. Wiirzler, F.M. de Souza Silva-Comar, Saulo Euclides Silva-Filho, Grosso do Sul & M.J.A. de Oliveira - **International Journal of Applied Research in Natural Products** (Jan. 2015).

100 - *Inhibitory Activity of Illicium Verum Extracts against Avian Viruses* - Mohammed S. Alhajj, Mahmood A. Qasem & Saud I. Al-Mufarrej - **Advances in Virology** (25 Jan. 2020).

Learn more about Coronaviruses (including SARS-COV-2) at:
https://theantiviraldiet.com/research-on-coronaviruses

Learn more about research on Diet and Phytotherapeutics at:
https://theantiviraldiet.com/research-on-diet-therapy-1

AVD the anti-viral diet
<u>SUMMARY OVERVIEW</u>

1. *Modern Scientific Research into Natural Anti-Virals and Immuno-Enhancing Chemicals has been Productive - it has shown that many of these are actually Dietary Ingredients*

2. *There is High Safety and Low Toxicity associated with Dietary Ingredients when ingested at Recommended Levels - Dietary Anti-Virals are therefore a Viable Option*

3. *There are Numerous Viral Threats and Viral Illnesses to which we have No Known Cure - Treatment Options, even Dietary, are an Important Consideration for All*

4. *An Anti-Viral Diet is one which focuses on Including a Number of Dietary Ingredients that Scientific Research does confirm have Anti-Viral & Immuno-Enhancing Effects*

5. *Candidates for Anti-Viral Ingredients in such a Diet are to be those which have the Most Corroborative Scientific Evidence*

6. *The Proposal of an 'Anti-Viral 5-a-Day' is being Recommended as a Minimum Requirement for an Anti-Viral Diet*

7. *The Anti-Viral Diet is a Dietary Proposal and is Not Presented as a Dietary Cure*

theantiviraldiet.com

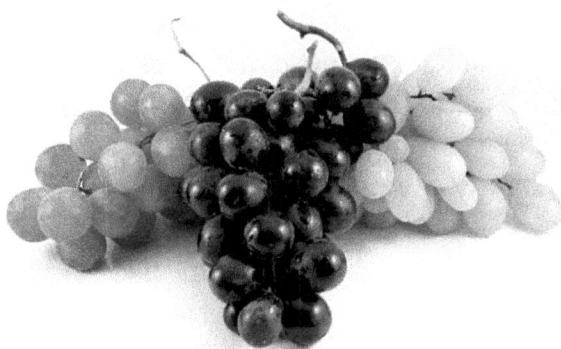

AN **AFTERWORD** BY THE AUTHOR

NO SINGLE INDIVIDUAL can be the author of an 'Anti-Viral Diet'. That is my opinion. If I have attached my name to this publication, it is so that all criticisms and questions regarding this project will be directed to and against me, and not levelled at the researchers from whose work I have drawn many of my own conclusions. If any of my inferences or suppositions are deemed to have gone beyond the facts or evidence in any way – even though I have done my best to avoid doing that, every step of the way – then it is I who am responsible for this, not the incredible pantheon of scientists who have opened up to us the knowledge of diet, nutrition, plant chemicals, microbiology, viruses, infectious diseases and more than we could ever have imagined knowing about one hundred years ago.

However, even though this volume has been an attempt to present a scientific hypothesis with a quantity of evidence that goes some distance toward supporting it, I am aware of how personal is this report on scientific findings – how much it is coloured by my own beliefs and opinions. Even though I have done my best to be as objective as possible in the appraisal of research data – and I have tried to be careful not to draw wider conclusions than those that results allow – nonetheless as a *single individual* authoring this study, it is more biased by one person's opinions than if it had been compiled and composed by a body of researchers. That is one reason why 'The Science Behind **AVD**' – the sequel to this volume – is written by an entire group of scientists from differing areas of expertise, thus providing a multiplicity of corroborative perspectives.

One thing that I must explain – before any insult is taken – is why I have not included the academic titles of any of the researchers within citations. This has not been out of a lack of respect, but because I want all of the research cited in this study to be considered on the same level, without the honours or seniority of one scientist giving us more belief in the credibility of their labours than in that of any students or junior academics.

Science cares not for age or positions - only for facts, analysis and conclusions. Hopefully I have caused no-one any offence.

This 'diet' is open to many more criticisms, one of which I can already hear quite distinctly - and that is: how come some ingredients included are solitary compounds, clearly defined, while others are food ingredients which contain a number of different chemicals within them? I did not think ill of making that choice because *this* is only the *first stage* in considering such a diet seriously. Later stages may lead to more precise levels of distinction between components - ultimately essential as some of the ingredients contain several bioactive constituents, each of which requires an individual appraisal.

The creation of a complete and reliable *anti-viral diet* truly requires a team of hundreds of nutritional and dietary scientists, working in collaboration with leading lights from many other relevant disciplines - all of them committed to such a project for as much time as it takes to come to full fruition. I would urge all countries of the world to come together and work in alignment with each other in order to accomplish such an admirable goal. For *if it is possible* that viruses and viral illnesses may one day all be deterred by diet alone, then I think that is a valuable and worthy 'science project' to pursue - one that can have an impact on the health and well-being of mankind from the day that it is discovered and as long as it is followed.

All that I have attempted to do here, has been to take one step in the right direction - though I may have tripped and stumbled in numberless places. The only thing that I feel confident about in this task, is that I have given *some definition* to what may be expected of an anti-viral diet, though only the perseverance of scientists can make it a reality. My time and resources were limited, but with the right team of researchers behind it and with the energy and determination to achieve what appears to be within our reach, I believe that an effective and invaluable Anti-Viral Diet might become a reality for us, even in time to ease the current crisis. **Edouard d'Araille**

MEDICAL DISCLAIMER

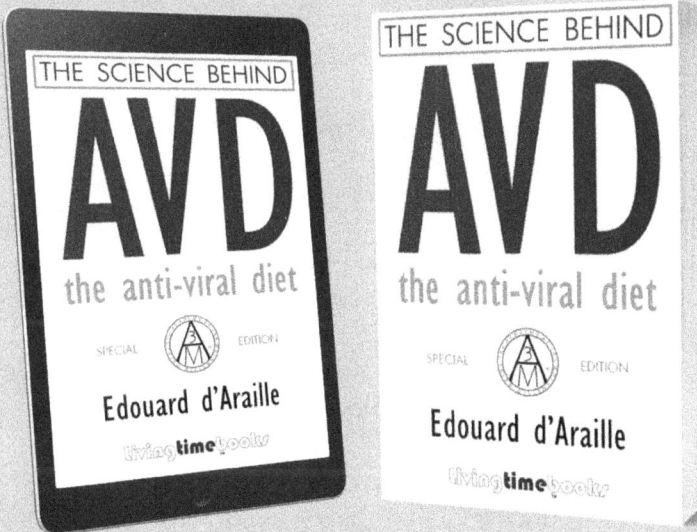

Other Works by
Edouard d'Araille

NON-FICTION
*The Cosmic Mirror - Being
Life, Art and the Cinema of
Six Dimensions* (Philosophy)
*Pre-Posthumous Notes of
an Anti-Critic* (Collected Essays)
Brave New Life (2021)

TRANSLATION
Adapa's Ascent - The First Story
(from the Akkadian & Sumerian)
Lafcadio Hearn: A Biographical Sketch
(from the German of Stefan Zweig)
*In the Temple of Dreams: The Writer on
the Screen* (Lectures, from the French
of Alain Robbe-Grillet *et alia*)

FICTION
FEATURES IN
Future Past and Other Premonitions
(Story Anthology)
The Immortals (Story Anthology)
The Vanishment (Story Anthology)
AUTHOR OF
Black Cab & Other Movies
(Story Anthology)
Crimes Past Murder in America (Novel)
Crime &nd Fortune (Part I)

POETRY
Poesia Nueva
In a Short Space of Time
Words Can't Hold ...
Ground Zero: 00/00/00
Ghetto Estate
WMD Words of Mass Destruction
Je Suis Poëte

www.A3M.uk

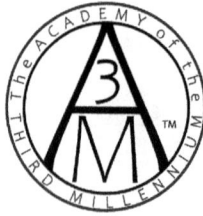

Knowledge is for Everyone

*A Wise Man should consider
that Health is the Greatest
of Human Blessings.*

HIPPOCRATES

Published by

living**time**books
TM

This Publication is set in
Luz Sans Book Typeface

www.ingramcontent.com/pod-product-compliance
Lightning Source LLC
Chambersburg PA
CBHW071018280326
41935CB00011B/1400